The Sickled Cell

FROM MYTHS TO MOLECULES

The Sickled Cell

FROM MYTHS
TO MOLECULES

Stuart J. Edelstein

Harvard University Press
Cambridge, Massachusetts
London, England   1986

This book is printed on acid-free paper, and
its binding materials have been chosen
for strength and durability.

Library of Congress Cataloging-in-Publication Data

Edelstein, Stuart J.
  The sickled cell.

  Bibliography: p.
  Includes index.
  1. Sickle cell anemia. 2. Sickle cell anemia—Africa. I. Title. [DNLM: 1.
Anemia, Sickle Cell. 2. Health Services, Indigenous—Africa. WH 170 E21s]
RC641.7.S5E34 1986   614.5'91527   86-2003
ISBN 0-674-80737-5 (alk. paper)

For Lynn, Jenny, and Dan

PREFACE

On my last trip to Nigeria I was in an Igbo village talking with a traditional healer about my interest in the anemia caused by sickling red blood cells. After I explained what was meant by anemia and sickling, he said that he understood anemia because traditional healers recognized such a condition, which they called "water in the blood." This novel way of characterizing anemia was instructive to me. Western scientists know that a low blood count is due to inadequate production of blood cells, but an observer unaware of the underlying mechanism might just as logically deduce that some defect allowed excess water into the blood. In Africa I frequently encountered new ways of looking at matters that were familiar to me, and I observed startling rituals for healing that seem to have arisen in response to these views.

One such practice was the amputation of the last bone of the left little finger of certain children identified as "repeater children," who, it was believed, died young only to be reborn to the same parents. Ritual amputation was the healer's method of inducing the child to "stay." A possible connection between repeater children and sickle cell anemia—a disease which can cause painful swelling of the joints of the fingers, sometimes interfering with the development of the hand and often leading to early death—had been suggested in the scientific literature, but no one has systematically explored this possibility. I decided to undertake this anthropological investigation during my field work in Africa, as an adjunct to my ongoing laboratory research into the molecular basis of sickling.

Eventually I became convinced that a book presenting these two aspects of sickle cell anemia—the anthropological and the molecular—might serve a useful purpose, particularly if it stimulates fresh approaches to the development of a safe and effective antisickling agent. Such an agent has remained elusive, despite our knowledge of almost all of the molecular details of sickling. By comparison, our knowledge of this disease in its original African setting is sparse; yet the natural products used in traditional African medicine may very well hold the secret to a major advance in treatment. It is my hope that this book will kindle an interest in research into those possibilities.

Sickle cell anemia originated in the African tropics, where the incidence is still very high—approximately one out of every fifty newborns in certain regions. My own field work began with the Igbos, a large ethnic group of southeastern Nigeria. Some of their traditions are introduced in Chapter 1, especially the fascinating concept of *ogbanje*, or repeater children, which was the focus of my research. To place the cultural aspects of sickling in their biological context, however, I first present in Chapter 2 an overview of late primate evolution, particularly as it appears in relation to the hemoglobin molecule. In Chapter 3 I examine the precise estimates that can be made concerning the timing and incidence of the sickle mutation. These estimates attempt to balance the disadvantages of the handicaps caused by sickle cell anemia against the slight advantage the mutation confers in the form of resistance to malaria. Then, a detailed examination of the *ogbanje* children among the Igbo is presented in Chapter 4, along with a description of the similar *àbikú* concept among their Nigerian neighbors, the Yoruba. A survey of related concepts among other ethnic groups across the African tropics reveals that the idea of repeater children is pervasive in West Africa. Although a one-to-one relation between *ogbanje* and sickling could not be demonstrated, there is suggestive evidence for a historical connection.

While clear relations cannot always be established in the cultural domain, precise descriptions can be achieved for molecules. The second half of the book is devoted to the details of the molecular aspects of sickling. In Chapter 5 the fundamental features of the mutation in DNA that changes hemoglobin to the sickling form are presented, with a discussion of the impact of these discoveries for molecular biology. The surprisingly intricate details of the sickle fibers and how they distort red cells are discussed in Chapter 6. Practical problems facing the diagnosis and treatment of sickling are then explored, with aspects concerning DNA presented in Chapter 7 and strategies aimed at altering the hemoglobin or other cellular components considered in Chapter 8. Following this sequence of topics from the cultural to the molecular, the book circles back to Africa in the last chapter to consider possible antisickling approaches derived from traditional African medicine.

The final form of this book emerged after a series of earlier versions that were read and critiqued by six colleagues to whom I am greatly indebted: Drs. H. F. Bunn, W. A. Eaton, M. Goossens, L. C. Jackson, N. Neaher, and C. Poyart. Various drafts were also read by T. Auld, L. Edelstein, and M. Rozycki, who offered valuable comments on questions of clarity and style. I also wish to express my thanks for helpful discussions on various topics considered here to C. Acquaye, B. Alter, R. Benesch, R. E. Benesch, L. Benjamin, J. Bernard, M. Bessis, Y. Beuzard, R. M. Bookchin, J. Brady, S. Charache, R. H. Crepeau, G. Dykes, F. Ferrone, F. Galacteros, M.-C. Garel, J. Hercules, J. Hofrichter, W. Love, B. Lubin, B. Magdoff-Fairchild, C. T. Noguchi, R. N. Nagel, E. P. Orringer, J. Pagnier, D. Rodgers, J. Rosa, R. Rosa, E. F. Roth, A. N. Schechter, G. Serjeant, I. Stevenson, M. H. Steinberg, W. Soyinka, F. Udekwu, J. A. Walder, G. D. Webb, and S. Wodak.

I am most grateful to the many individuals whose help and cooperation I received during my field work in Africa, especially the *ogbanje* children and their families. My appreciation for their varied assistance during that phase of my research also goes to C. Ani, R. G. Armstrong, R. Cabannes, O. Ebohon, N. Ibekwe, W. N. Kaine, B. Kalu, J. Lonsdorfer, J. Ndour, G. O. Obi, F. Ogah, P. Onwuka, P. Onyekelu, Z. Sossah, R. N. Tagbo, D. Udeji, and S. Wenger. I am particularly indebted to I. Stevenson for encouraging me to embark on field work in Nigeria and for sharing his resources with me. The Institute for African Studies, University of Ibadan, granted me an Associate Membership and access to their facilities, which I gratefully acknowledge.

Most of the final writing of this book was carried out during a sabbatical year (1984-1985) in France, where I enjoyed the hospitality and support of J. Rosa, Y. Beuzard, M. Goossens, and C. Poyart. I would also like to thank the Fogerty Center, NIH, for granting me a Senior International Fellowship during that time.

Harvard University Press's Editor for Science and Medicine, Howard Boyer, participated in both the inception and the realization of this project and offered valuable suggestions on organization. Senior Editor Susan Wallace skillfully edited the final manuscript.

For kindly providing or helping in the preparation of illustrations I thank Drs. O. Akinyanju, C. Barrière, M. Bessis, J. S. Cohen, R. H. Crepeau, G. Dykes, W. A. Eaton, M. E. Fabry, Y. W. Kan, F. I. D. Konotey-Ahulu, N. Neaher, W. Noon, D. Rodgers, G. Serjeant, T. Shaw, M. Szalay, J. Telford, A. Tunis, L. van Deenen, and J. J. Yunis.

And finally, I wish to acknowledge a great debt to my family for encouraging me in these pursuits and for tolerating my absences during the field work in Africa and my preoccupations during writing periods.

S. J. E.
May 1986

CONTENTS

The Sickled Cell

FROM MYTHS TO MOLECULES

CHAPTER 1

THE SICKLE
OF AFRICA

Ancient philosophers have said that even so simple an object as a grain of sand can, when thoroughly contemplated, reveal the workings of the universe. They probably had in mind a purely mental process, perhaps a cross-legged yogi sitting Buddha-like, locked in some intriguing inner exploration. For scientists today, a grain of sand might still be a gateway to the mysteries of the universe, but powerful microscopes and other sophisticated instruments would be used to study its structure and chemical properties. The geological history of the earth might be invoked to explain sand in its cosmic setting, and the tools of the linguist might be employed to trace the origins of the word "sand" itself. As though searching for footprints in the sands of time, we might eventually be led into an exploration of the human imagination, where sand can become a powerful metaphor in the hands of a gifted poet.

For most scientists, their particular subjects are so specialized, their instruments so complex, the information they need to keep current so voluminous, that it has become increasingly difficult to step outside the confines of their special interest and try to place it in a broader context. But some subjects seem to lend themselves to just such an expanded view. The sickled cell, with its distribution among the varied peoples of tropical Africa, is a particularly powerful grain of sand that leads naturally into broader considerations of evolution and culture. However, these topics have been relatively neglected, compared with the molecular and cellular aspects of sickling—at least in part because of an inherent complexity that can never be mastered as fully as precise chemical details.[1] Nevertheless, during the last decade, while analyzing the molecular interactions within sickled cells in my laboratory, I became curious about, and began to investigate, the cultural aspects of sickling. Eventually, from a series of trips to Africa to study the impact of sickling in its original setting, some intriguing patterns began to emerge. Although far from complete, these findings, together with information recently brought to light by other investigators, dramatically illustrate the potential impact of the simplest type of genetic mutation on the evolution of a society's myths and traditions. This book explores these implications, in the hope that a broader knowledge of sickle cell anemia in its natural setting might provide insights into the disease that would influence the development of antisickling agents and other treatments. Further awareness of the African experience, particularly the traditional African response to sickle cell anemia, will also be very important in facilitating acceptance of any new treatment that scientists might devise.

In this first chapter, the essentials of the sickling process will be sketched and some generalities about African languages and cultures formulated, leading to discussion of the special mixture of tradition and innovation one finds in contemporary Nigeria. The chapter ends with a glimpse of the remarkable Igbo "repeater children," who exhibit some intriguing cultural links to sickle cell disease.[2] Subsequent chapters will explore specific aspects of sickling, from the general principles of evolution that led to its proliferation, to specific details of the atomic interactions responsible for these misshapen cells. And finally, we will discuss the promise of several new approaches to the treatment of sickle cell anemia.

The introduction of the word "sickle" goes back to 1910, when J. B. Herrick, a Chicago physician, was examining the blood of an anemic black student from the West Indies. Looking through his microscope, Herrick was startled to see not the usual rounded red blood cells but rather "peculiar elongated and sickle-shaped" cells.[3] Since then, scientists have discovered that sickling occurs only when there is a certain mutation in the gene that specifies a part of hemoglobin.(the protein in red blood cells responsible for taking up oxygen in the lungs and transporting it to the rest of the body). A change in just one of the smallest building blocks of the gene leads to a minor alteration in this complex protein, but one which nevertheless causes the hemoglobin molecules to stick to one another and form fibers that distort the red blood cells into their characteristic sickle shape (Fig. 1.1). The mutant form of he- moglobin is known as sickle hemoglobin, or more simply hemo- globin S.

In spite of our wealth of knowledge about the sickling process, researchers have not yet been able to develop a general treatment for the disease that sickling causes, namely, sickle cell anemia. The problem is especially acute because of the relatively large numbers of people afflicted. Whereas most genetic diseases are

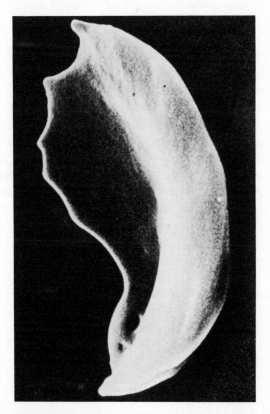

Figure 1.1. A sickled cell as seen in the scanning electron microscope. The sickled cell is about 10 microns across (1 micron = one-millionth of a meter). (From M. Bessis.)

limited to a very few cases, the population of individuals with sickling cells is high because carriers of the gene—those who inherit the sickle hemoglobin gene from just one parent and a normal hemoglobin gene from the other parent—appear to have a slight resistance to malaria. As a result of this genetic advantage that carriers have over noncarriers, in those regions of Africa infested with malaria more and more carriers have survived in each generation over thousands of years. Today, in certain regions of Africa, 20–30% of the population are carriers. Carriers are effectively free of the symptoms of sickle cell anemia; the normal gene keeps the red blood cells from sickling. But children produced from the union of two carriers have one chance in four of inheriting the sickle gene from *both* parents. Lacking a normal gene to protect them, these individuals will develop sickle cell anemia with its associated problems in blood circulation.

Sickled cells are fragile and do not live as long in the blood stream as normal cells, which have a life span of about 120 days. Because of the much shorter life of sickled cells, as short as 30 days in some cases, individuals with sickling cells have difficulty keeping up their red blood cell production; the result is anemia. More serious than anemia for these individuals, however, are the various blockages that can occur in the blood stream. Sickled cells are more rigid than normal cells. Consequently, their passage through the tiny capillaries that connect veins to arteries can be hindered to such an extent that blood flow is clogged. Ironically, anemia may actually help to reduce the pain and damage caused by clogging; if more cells were present, blockages in the capillaries would occur more readily and have more serious consequences.

Sickle cell anemia makes its presence known during the first year after birth and is likely to lead to a difficult childhood and uncertain prospects for survival into adulthood. In the United States the average life expectancy for an individual with sickle cell anemia is currently 20 years and is increasing. Under less favorable medical conditions, as in many parts of Africa, life expectancy is much shorter. A total of about 50,000 people with sickle cell anemia live in the United States today, whereas in Africa this number of infants with sickle cell anemia may be born every year.

Although traces of sickling can be found throughout the African continent, individuals who carry the sickle mutation live principally in the band of tropical forest which crosses equatorial Africa (Fig. 1.2). Within these limits is a region of astounding size and diversity. The casual visitor to Africa who travels from coast to coast by air has difficulty grasping the dimensions of this area and the great ocean of humanity welling below. The distance from Dakar at the western edge of Africa to Nairobi near the east-

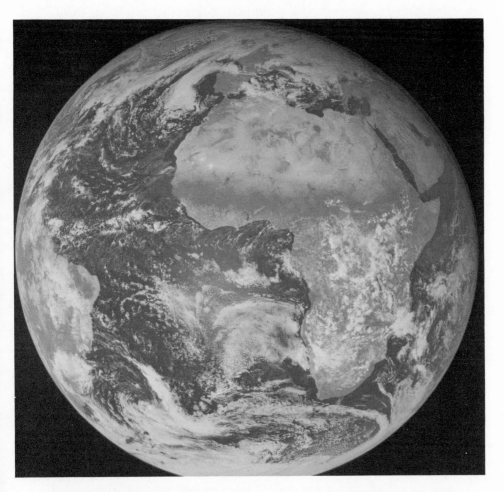

Figure 1.2. Africa, the sickle-shaped continent, as viewed from space. The long dimension of the African continent is about 10,000 kilometers. The tropics form a belt across the center of the continent. (From National Remote Sensing Centre, Farnborough, England.)

ern edge is greater than the distance across the Atlantic from New York to London.

The superficial similarities of ethnic groups in tropical Africa mask an incredible diversity of languages and traditions. Hundreds of distinct languages are spoken across this region. As measured by linguistic standards, languages that are as different as Sanskrit and English are sometimes spoken by neighboring peoples. The Hausa and Igbo peoples of Nigeria fit this description. In the classification which divides African languages into four great phyla, Hausa is placed in the phylum that includes the Semitic languages, such as Arabic and Hebrew. Igbo belongs to the phylum with the other Niger-Congo languages. Linguistic measures of the relatedness of these languages indicate that they have been independent thousands of years, with numerous and often lengthy migrations accounting for the current arrangement of ethnic groups.[4]

A distinctive feature of the languages in this region is that they were, with few exceptions, never written. Apart from a limited number such as Wolof and Peul in West Africa, for which transcriptions were made with the arabic alphabet in the eighteenth century, it was only with the arrival of European visitors at the end of the last century that efforts on a large scale were made to apply alphabets to the languages. In some societies pictograms were in use, as in the case of the pictorial language of the Igbo called *nsibidi,* and such efforts might have developed into a written language along the lines of Chinese characters or Egyptian hieroglyphics had not the colonial powers arrived to introduce their forms of literacy.

Another feature of most African languages, and one which complicates their study by Americans and Europeans, is tonality—words that are spelled the same have different meanings, depending on the pitch of the syllables. Among the few notable exceptions are the Wolof and Serer languages at the western extremity of the African tropics and Swahili at the eastern extremity. Fula, the language of the Fulani, one of the most migratory peoples of Africa, is also nontonal. For serious investigators of African culture, the tonal languages have often presented a particularly formidable barrier. Indeed, tonality may be the dominant factor in mastery of an African language. According to W. E. Welmers, an expert in African linguistics:

Many of the younger generation of investigators have been willing to face this fact, but even among them the attitude is all too common that they would prefer to master the consonants and vowels, most of the grammar, and a great deal of vocabulary, and then they will tackle the supposedly knotty problem of tone. Apart from the weightier considerations of the possible functions of tone in a language, there is one intensely practical reason why this procedure is virtually doomed to failure. By the time the investigator decides to settle down and learn something about tone, the people from whom he has been learning the language will already have decided long since that he will never pronounce their language accurately. They will have given up correcting him, and they will utterly fail to comprehend what he is after now. To the native speaker of a tone language, tone is just as basic a part of his speech as consonants and vowels; if no progress is made in the aspect of pronunciation at first, there is no reason to expect that any improvement will be made later.[5]

The confusions that can result from neglecting tone are nearly limitless; to cite just one example, in the Igbo language *ényi* is elephant and *ényì* is friend. The accent aigu, *é*, indicates a high tone, while the accent grave, *è*, indicates a low tone. A midtone is also employed, designated by a vertical accent, as at the end of *àbúọ̀* (the Igbo word for "two"). In sentences, a downward progression of successive tones is superimposed on the tones of the individual words in what is called a terracing of tones that commonly leads to many more than three distinct tones in a single sentence. For example, if tones are indicated under the syllables of a sentence by letters from *a* to *z*, where *a* is the highest tone of the sentence and *z* is the lowest, the sentence for "my brother and his teacher came to our house" would be described:

> *nwa nne m na onye nkuzi ya byara ulo anyi.*
>
> a a b b z c c c c c d   z z e f g g

In this case, the trained ear can detect eight distinct tones.

African languages, like those of indigenous societies from other parts of the world, are extremely rich in names for all of the objects in their environments. Observers have emphasized the advanced taxonomical dexterity of many African languages, including, for example, an ethno-botanical list of about 8,000 terms collected from Gabon, the western-most nation of continental Africa traversed by the equator. Moreover, the knowledge is not limited to experts, as noted in E. S. Bowen's recollection of experiences among the Tiv, the neighbors of the Igbo to the northeast: "I found myself in a place where every plant, wild or cultivated, had a name and use and where every man, woman and child knew literally hundreds of plants."[6]

In contrast to the specificity of certain categories of descriptive nouns, abstract concepts in most African languages are not expressed in ways that correspond to expressions in most European languages. One obstacle to the study of Igbo notions of the self or the individual, for example, arises from the fact that in the Igbo language the verb "to be" can be expressed in three different ways, none of which would be suitable for translating Hamlet's soliloquy. Perhaps this situation reflects a sense of being that is so innately integrated with the environment that it requires no designation.

A strength of African languages typical of ancient societies concerns their facility for designating relationships. Since all African ethnic groups have strong traditions of kinship, particularly in regard to marriage, it is not surprising that many of their languages provide a richer vocabulary of pronouns and terms for relatives than can be found in English. In the case of Nama, one of the Hottentot languages, there are 10 ways to say "we," depending on various combinations of "I" with others, male or female, singular or plural, and second or third person. Since similar distinctions apply to the translation of our word "they," the simple sentence "We gave it to them" could be translated in 60 different ways.[7]

While every ethnic group in Africa has an extensive oral tradition, the absence of written historical records limits the availability of information about the past. History is recorded in the minds of the elders and passed along from generation to generation, and formidable efforts are required of scholars who wish to obtain such oral histories. More readily accessible are the travel accounts of the early European visitors, the more recent writings of anthropologists (usually in the language of the colonial power in the area studied), and, most recently, writings of Africans educated in a European language, mainly English or French.

Differences attributed to national style were at one time perceived in the various approaches to African studies. French scholars tended to orient their inquiries around the mythology of the

ethnic groups they studied, in order to learn how people con-
ceived of themselves in relation to their world and the cosmos.
English scholars tended to emphasize everyday activities and
their ritualistic aspects. In recent years distinctions between what
was once summarized as "the French emphasis on cosmology and
the British concern with ritual" have become less meaningful, as
scholars writing in both languages have tackled a broad range of
subjects and as more and more "pragmatic" Americans have entered African studies.[8] Nevertheless, it is instructive to note how
deep-seated are certain stereotypes typically applied to distinguish between the English and the French, not just in African
studies but in almost every area of inquiry. For example, the
English scientific hero of the nineteenth century, Charles Darwin,
was a naturalist in the tradition of Francis Bacon—an observer,
collector, and organizer of information, who brought this empirical approach to a high point with his theory of evolution through
natural selection. For the same period, the French scientific hero
was Louis Pasteur, an experimentalist in the tradition of René
Déscartes. Pasteur was a laboratory scientist who applied tightly
controlled logic to his investigations in chemistry, microbiology,
and immunology. For these and other related reasons, labels such
as the "empirical" English and the "rational" French have been
widely used to generalize about two peoples that are in fact extremely similar compared with the diversity among African ethnic groups.

The point I wish to make here is that whether or not such distinctions between the English and the French are valid, we have
sufficiently rich impressions to permit us to find many arguments
for or against such generalities. In contrast, the impressions generally held about different African ethnic groups are overly homogeneous—the diversity of African peoples is only dimly perceived.
However, a first-hand observer soon begins to notice many distinguishing characteristics of African ethnic groups. For example,
the two major ethnic groups of southern Nigeria, the Yoruba and
the Igbo, are by a number of criteria more different than any two
major nationalities of Western Europe. Recognizing significant
differences within a framework of similarities is one of the major
challenges facing any comprehensive effort to understand African
culture.

Focusing on just one country, Nigeria, we confront a diversity that represents a microcosm for all of Africa. Nigeria, which occupies an area one-third larger than the state of Texas, bulges with a population conservatively estimated by the United Nations to be 80 million. The most populous African country, Nigeria also has one of the highest incidences of carriers of the sickle mutation. Among the Yoruba and the Igbo, sickle carriers make up approximately 25% of the population. Nigeria is a dynamic, ebullient, boisterous country possessing such striking contrasts between the modern and the ancient that my extensive reading only partially prepared me for a visit. The images of Africa found in literary sources capture certain details, but for me the overwhelming sensation upon arrival was the indescribably sweet aroma of lush tropical vegetation, mixed in more populated areas with the smells of cooking fires and the odors of animals and people, all borne on waves of humid air accompanied by the rhythms of the ever present Calypso-like music from radios and tape recorders.

For the visitor to Nigeria, the first stop is always the large and modern Murtala Mohammed International Airport near Lagos (Fig. 1.3), but travels to the interior originate at the more modest national airport. At departure time, the airport gate is opened, the plane is pointed to, and the would-be passengers take off in a sprint. Since the best way to ensure having a seat on the plane is to be sitting in it, running to the plane is a tradition in Nigeria that has not disappeared, even with the advent of more reliable booking practices. My years of running were put to a rare practical use as I was one of the first to occupy a seat. My first trip to Enugu was thus assured. The southeastern part of Nigeria is the homeland of the Igbo, and Enugu was briefly the capital of the ill-fated attempt by the Igbo and other less populous groups of this region to create the independent state of Biafra in 1967. Although Enugu was quickly conquered by Federal Nigerian troops, portions of Biafra to the south held out longer.

After achieving its independence from England in 1960, Nigeria was governed by democratic rule in an effort to bring harmony to the new nation, but a military government was established by *coup d'état* in 1965. A succession of military governments continued through the Biafra period, or what is referred to outside Igboland as the Nigerian Civil War. The military leadership, under a plan initiated by Brigadier Murtala Mohammed,

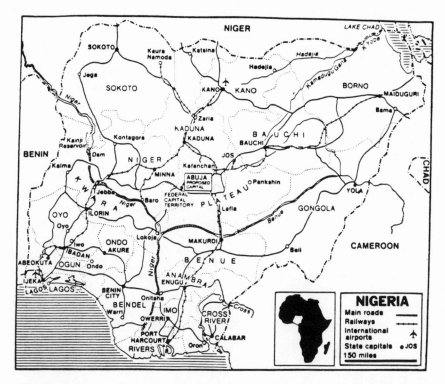

Figure 1.3. Map of Nigeria. The Igbo live mainly in the states of Anambra and Imo.

returned the country to civilian control in 1979. Shehu Shagari, a member of the major northern ethnic group, the Hausa, was elected President. He appeared to have achieved some success in balancing the rivalries of the major ethnic groups, principally by distributing oil wealth to the 19 small states into which the country had been divided. The Igbo live mainly in two states, Anambra and Imo. Enugu is the capital of Anambra State.

Shagari was re-elected President in the fall of 1983. However, his second term was brought to an early termination with a *coup d'état* on December 31, 1983, that returned the military to power once again. The military cited rigging of the recent election, a precarious economy, and, especially, high levels of corruption to justify its action. According to some reports, bribery on a large scale permeated all levels of Nigerian government. A major oil-producing country, Nigeria relied heavily on oil income to finance the importation of large quantities of food, and it neglected internal agriculture. With the drop in oil prices that preceded the 1983 coup, serious food shortages and other hardships threatened. The suspension of one of the few remaining democracies among the nations of Africa (and what had been the largest) dramatizes the difficulty of progressing from a traditional society to a freely elected central government, particularly when a number of distinct ethnic groups are involved.

While certain peoples of Nigeria have a tradition of empires and royalty, the Igbo have preferred decentralized authority. As a result, cities such as Enugu are relatively young and lack the history of a place such as Benin City to the west, where the court of the Obi has been flourishing for centuries. It was first described in Europe by Portuguese sailors in the 1400s. The arrival of the Portuguese marked the beginning of a mutual fascination between Europeans and Africans. The Portuguese carried back to their homeland sketches and written accounts of the exotic rulers they had seen, and the Obi's metalsmiths captured the likenesses of the Portuguese in bronze statues. Much later, these statues and many other exquisite examples of Benin bronze objects found their way to Europe, when the court of the Obi was pillaged by British soldiers in 1897.

The Igbo preference for small villages and decentralized authority is still readily apparent to the visitor. Leaving Enugu with its tall Presidential Hotel—complete with elevators, a swimming pool, and a TELEX machine—to head south along a modern divided highway, one soon encounters dirt roads that lead off into the forest. After some distance the dirt road may narrow to a footpath and at the end of the path may be found a remote village where the developments of the modernized world have made little impact. On such a journey I feel that I am traveling back in time to glimpse the human situation as it must have been in its infancy—beautifully simple, but extremely vulnerable.

The beauty comes from a near-perfect integration of the inhabitants with their environment, living off the land which provides the farms for growing yams and cassava. Small plots are slashed and burned out of the forest for planting and after several years are allowed to return to their natural state while the farming activities move elsewhere. The success of this activity is demonstrated by population densities of 1,000 per square mile in some areas, among the highest in the world for rural areas subsisting on root crops raised by hoe farming.[9] At a deeper level, one senses a beauty in their harmonious animist vision of the world and their place in it. In the animist perspective, all activities are the consequence of spiritual beings and entities. Thus, every aspect of life is part of a drama of natural forces dominated by spirits and deceased ancestors interceding to influence the application of these forces, be it for better crops or more children.

Many of the early missionaries to Africa found little redeeming merit in the African culture, however, and saw their own role as educating these uninformed peoples in both secular and religious matters, while weaning them away from their pagan practices. The missionaries were shocked, for example, by the Igbo belief that the birth of twins was an abomination to be resolved by abandoning newborn twins in the bush. While striking us as blatantly inhuman, in the Igbo experience mothers may have rarely been able to nurture twins; the effort often resulted in the deaths of all three. Moreover, in Igbo society the birth of twins was viewed as the twins' misfortune; the mother should not have to choose one over the other in order to rectify the problem. As will be discussed in a later chapter, similar attitudes are currently encountered in African societies plagued by high infant mortalities; the result is the development of strategies that delay bonding by the mother until evidence appears that the child is going to "stay." In this way maternal anguish over the premature death of an infant may be lessened. The missionaries succeeded in eliminating twin infanticide, but their revulsion at such practices may have led to a lack of appreciation of other, more positive qualities in the Igbo culture.

As in many indigenous societies, feats of considerable insight and skill were produced before contact with European civilization—for the Igbos, most notably, in metalwork. Excavations in Igbo territory carried out under the direction of Thurstan Shaw have unearthed many bronze objects of striking composition and remarkable craftsmanship. The most famous is a foot-high water pot standing on its own pedestal and enclosed by intricate, simulated ropework (Fig. 1.4). The thousand-year-old pot was prepared by "lost wax" bronze casting, probably in several stages.

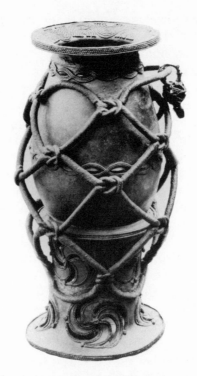

Figure 1.4. Bronze water pot from the excavations at Igbo-Ukwu. (From the National Museum, Lagos, Nigeria. Photographed by D. Simmonds.)

Referring to accomplishments such as this and others in plant cultivation, animal domestication, pottery, and herbal medicine initiated in neolithic cultures, Claude Lévi-Strauss has perceived the underlying activities that such achievements require:

> Each of these techniques assumes centuries of active and methodical observation, of bold hypotheses tested by means of endlessly repeated experiments ... There is no doubt that all these achievements require a genuinely scientific attitude, sustained and watchful interest and a desire for knowledge for its own sake. For only a small proportion of observations and experiments (which must be assumed to have been primarily inspired by a desire for knowledge) could have yielded practical and immediate results.[10]

According to Lévi-Strauss, a form of scientific activity has existed since the earliest so-called primitive societies. However, this older science was not necessarily a forerunner or step on the way to the modern scientific method, but rather an alternative or parallel form that is more intuitive and mythic, involving small innovations in existing structures—much like the development of myths themselves, or language. Existing forms are used and reused in various ways without regard to singularity of purpose, so that enterprises have a "second-hand" character. In the original French edition of his book *The Savage Mind*, Lévi-Strauss used the word "bricolage" to characterize this alternative form of scientific development. "Bricolage" means a patchwork construction, made by a reworking or "do-it-yourself" activity.

It is interesting to note that the word "bricolage" has also been used by the French biologist François Jacob to characterize evolution. In an important sense, both biological organisms and traditional cultures are limited to operating within a framework of existing structures that can only change in small steps. Thus, the Igbo metalsmiths mastered an evolutionary approach, whereas the technical accomplishments of engineers in our North Atlantic culture often involve innovations that depart radically from previous forms or concepts. As summarized by Jacob,

> First . . . the engineer works according to a preconceived plan. Second, an engineer who prepares a new structure does not necessarily work from older ones. The electric bulb does not derive from the candle, nor does the jet engine descend from the internal combustion engine. To produce something new, the engineer has at his disposal original blueprints drawn for that particular occasion, materials and machines specially prepared for that task. Finally, the objects thus produced de novo by the engineer, at least by the good engineer, reach the level of perfection made possible by the technology of the time. In contrast, evolution is far from perfection.[11]

Modern science has evolutionary elements in it as well, as every discovery builds on existing knowledge and techniques, but it differs fundamentally from mythic science in its orientation, since modern science is reductive: it "explains" relatively complex phenomena in terms of simpler principles. The property of matter is reduced to the characteristics of the electrons and the nucleus of the constituent atoms; biological phenomena are related to the properties of cells and their constituent molecules. Scientific knowledge progresses along a one-track, linear logic. Ultimately, nature is manipulated through actions directed at this fundamental level.

In this way nature is understood in terms of hidden causes that are generally too small to see without special devices. The microscope contributed greatly to the reductionist trend in biology, playing a role similar to that of the x-ray for physical sciences. Not having these reductive tools, the indigenous form of science found in Africa developed along integrative lines, based on external relationships and animist concepts of nature. Technical principles are thoroughly mixed with the mythology of the culture. The Igbo carefully put aside their best yams for planting the following season—a sound principle of plant breeding—but at the same time they offer sacrifices to *aha njoku* (the yam spirit) before planting. Thus, the logic is multi-track, or parallel, in the sense that events at two levels—material and spiritual—are pursued simultaneously, in contrast to the single track of modern science. The difficulty in studying the parallel science of indigenous cultures arises from this conglomeration of elements that are not easily separated into physical necessities and spiritual necessities. We will encounter this problem in our exploration of the relationship between certain traditional cultural practices and sickle cell disease.

In a certain sense, the great ideas of the nineteenth century, such as Darwin's theory of evolution in biology and Mendeleev's periodic table in chemistry, were the pinnacle of the nonreductive approach. Both ideas implied underlying mechanisms of some complexity, but Darwin had virtually no understanding of gene structure, nor had Mendeleev any conception of the atom. Of course, their achievements did not have the animist component of the mythic science practiced by traditional African cultures. Nevertheless, the workings of this mythic or integrative form of science will, I suspect, someday attract more interest as its possibilities for filling certain deficiencies in our currently dominant reductive science are appreciated. However, the opportunities for studying this "second" science are quickly vanishing, as places like Nigeria join the world of television and automobiles, participating in the global popular culture. This transition is inevitable, but efforts to collect information on many traditional cultures must be encouraged before the opportunities disappear entirely. Increasingly, in regions of Africa such as that of the Igbo, one follows the dirt road and the footpath to a small village, only to find a modern two-story house in the midst of the mud huts, a concrete testimony to the success of a village son or daughter. The current generation finds itself in a conflict between the traditional ways of village life and the modern international culture of the cities. In a few generations there may be no conflict, if the current trends of urbanization and westernization continue.

However, such philosophical issues do not impose themselves when one is in direct contact with the people in a traditional Igbo village. Practical realities dominate the landscape. As I mentioned, the old African ways have not only their beautifully simple side but an extremely vulnerable side as well. The vulnerability is all too apparent, especially in the realm of medical needs. From the remote villages, hospitals could be reached on foot in some cases, but the motivation is usually not present. Nigeria has a number of fine medical schools and training hospitals which serve increasing numbers of the population, but their patients come mostly from the cities. In the countryside, traditional ideas are still dominant and illness is not necessarily associated with medical causes in the sense familiar to us. Even death is not necessarily associated with bodily illness, but rather with a peculiarly African concept of complications of the soul.

As was explained by a French priest who has worked in Africa for more than 20 years, the Africans historically have neglected the physical type of medicine perfected in the technical societies, but have developed a "science of the soul" that went far beyond anything ever imagined in Europe or America. As a biochemist, I was not at all sure of what this priest had in mind by a "science of the soul," but as I learned more about African culture I began to perceive the grounds for his assertion. For example, an early study of death concepts among the Igbo notes the role of the hierarchy of supernatural entities, including God, *Chukwu*, the spirits of thunder and other forces, the spirits of land, and the ancestral or clan spirits. Then seven causes of death are listed with various specific examples, ranging from *onwutci*, a suitable end after a complete life fulfilling the destiny assigned by *Chukwu*, to less desirable deaths resulting from accidents triggered by spirits of misfortune or caused by violations of taboos. One type of death was limited to children who were called *ogbanje* (translated as "children who come and go," and who have also come to be known as the "repeater children").[12]

The identification of an *ogbanje* arose typically when a family had several children die soon after birth. In these circumstances, it was believed that a wicked soul had come repeatedly to the family to be born as a baby, only to leave soon after birth. Could this be the Igbo explanation of sickle cell anemia, in a family where both mother and father were carriers giving birth to several afflicted children in a row? It seems plausible, since in Africa, children with sickle cell disease often die very young. One of the consequences of sickle cell anemia is an extremely high sensitivity to infection in the first four years of life. In the United States, children diagnosed at birth as having sickle cell anemia are given penicillin at the first signs of possible infection to help survive this critical period. However, antibiotics are a relatively recent development and are still rarely used in rural Africa. Dehydration, a common consequence of diarrhea in Africa, would also worsen sickling.

That there might be a connection between *ogbanje* and sickle cell disease was discussed in 1976 by Elizabeth Isichei:

> Certain Igbo beliefs attempt to provide an explanation of imperfectly understood natural phenomena. An interesting example is the concept of the *ogbanje*. This is a wicked spirit which takes the form of a beautiful child. He is constantly reborn in a family, and constantly dies, tormenting the unfortunate parents. This may be an explanation of sickle-cell anemia, which is very common in Igboland: the children of distinctive physical appearance, dying in infancy or childhood, born to apparently healthy parents who are carriers of the sickle-cell trait.[13]

The possibility of a genetic disease playing a role in the *ogbanje* concept seemed eminently plausible, although one curious aspect concerned the notion that it would be a beautiful child. African concepts of beauty do not always coincide with those in Europe and America. For example, the current Western quest for slimness contrasts with the "fattening" that young Igbo women traditionally undergo before marriage. Some additional hints about African aesthetics might be derived from sculptures and masks, although the specific function of any object must be considered, since beauty is not always intended. However, for certain objects believed to depict beauty, such as the maiden spirit masks of the

Igbo (Fig. 1.5), there is an exaggeration of certain facial bones, especially those of the forehead. It could well be that the physical appearance of children with sickle cell disease conforms to Igbo notions of beauty, since a condition of skull bossing does sometimes accompany the disease (Fig. 1.6). Or perhaps all children are beautiful, especially when we are in sympathy for their deaths.

Leaving aside the subtle question of beauty, we can state with confidence that the existence of *ogbanje* children has long been a major concern to the Igbo. Mention of *ogbanjes* can be found in missionaries' journals dating from 1859, but only the most fragmentary studies on this subject have been carried out by anthropologists.[14] However, the subject of *ogbanje* has been given considerable attention by the Igbo novelist Chinua Achebe. His writings brilliantly bring to life the raw vitality of traditional Igbo society as it confronted the English colonialists and missionaries. In one of his most celebrated novels, *Things Fall Apart,* he captures the anguish of a mother, Ekwefi, confronted with an *ogbanje* experience:

> As she buried one child after another her sorrow gave way to despair and then to grim resignation. The birth of her children, which should be a woman's crowning glory, became for Ekwefi mere physical agony devoid of promise. The naming ceremony after seven market weeks became an empty ritual. Her deepening despair found expression in the names she gave her children. One of them was a pathetic cry, Onwumbiko—"Death, I implore you." But death took no notice; Onwumbiko died in his fifteenth month. The next child was a girl Ozoemena—"May it not happen again." She died in her eleventh month.

Later we learn that after Onwumbiko's death:

> The medicine man then ordered that there should be no mourning for the dead child. He brought out a sharp razor from the goatskin bag slung from his left shoulder and began to mutilate the child. Then he took it away to bury in the Evil Forest, holding it by the ankle and dragging it on the ground behind him. After such treatment it would think twice before coming again, unless it was one of the stubborn ones who returned, carrying the stamp of their mutilation—a missing finger or perhaps a dark line where the medicine man's razor had cut them.[15]

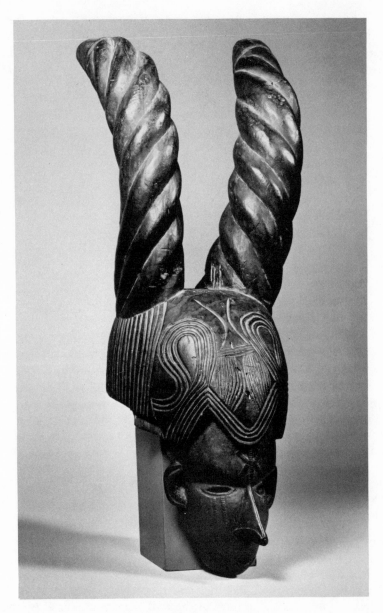

Figure 1.5. Igbo maiden spirit mask. (From the Herbert F. Johnson Museum of Art, Cornell University; gift of Katherine Kamaroff Goodman. Photographed by Jon Reis.)

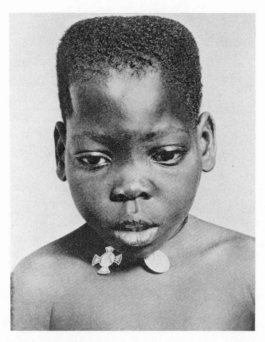

Figure 1.6. African child with bossed skull. (From Trowell, Raper, and Welbourn, 1957.)

The idea of a human drama based on the anguish caused by a malevolent, reincarnating spirit that frustrated efforts to create a normal family seemed to me to be too incredible a belief, even for peoples still living in a mythic world. Nevertheless, it was with vague images of *ogbanje* in mind that I began studying the Igbo. It was not difficult to find people willing to offer help—former Igbo students at Cornell University and faculty members at the University of Nigeria Teaching Hospital in Enugu. Actually making contact with people after arriving in Nigeria was a more difficult matter, since telephone communication is rarely possible and mail is slow. Soon after arriving in Nigeria for the first time, while Ian Stevenson, an American colleague, and I were trying to find a teacher who had offered assistance in Awgu (a small town about 30 miles south of Enugu), we entered a rural school on the outskirts of town. It was a typical African school, with one huge room, a corrugated tin roof, and walls completed only about halfway up to the roof. The students in their blue uniforms were unaccustomed to seeing Caucasians and shouted "Bèkéè, bèkéè!" ("white man") in enthusiastic excitement.

The principal greeted us and we promptly learned that the teacher we were seeking was not at the school. Nevertheless, the conversation was prolonged as a result of the inquisitiveness and hospitable qualities that are so highly developed among the Igbo. Visitors from Europe or America are often frustrated by the African style of accomplishing things—efficiency at times seems to be replaced by deliberate entanglements. I think this habit arose from the lack of a written language. The spoken word became the primary source of entertainment in a culture without print and other modern media, and conversation developed into an art form. A word that one hears throughout Africa is "palaver," derived from the Portuguese *palavra,* which means to have a lengthy conference or parley. Apparently even the Portuguese, the first Europeans to visit the Africans extensively, found this quality notable and left behind a word that they must have used frequently.

As the palaver with the rural school principal continued, the topic of *ogbanjes* came up and this led to the event that was to shape the future of my activities in Africa. The principal said, "I have several *ogbanjes* in my school," and called out a command to the children in Igbo. In a few seconds there were 10 children before us, boys and girls ranging in age from about 6 to 13. They were lovely children—shy, but wide-eyed—all looking perfectly fit (Fig. 1.7). The principal said something in Igbo and raised his left hand. As if in salute, the children followed suit, each raising the left hand. At that moment we could see that everything after the first joint of the little finger—the entire last bone—was missing.

As I stood before these children, I recalled the children in Achebe's narrative, born "carrying the stamp of their mutilation" by a medicine man on the corpse of a deceased sibling believed to be an *ogbanje.* I realized that a considerable effort would be needed to learn from these families their various stories. I felt a sense of awe and rare privilege at having stepped so deeply into the living world of a traditional African society. I also began thinking about sickling cells and the series of events—from mutation to migration—that led to a major genetic disease and may have triggered a new mythology. However, as with many subtle

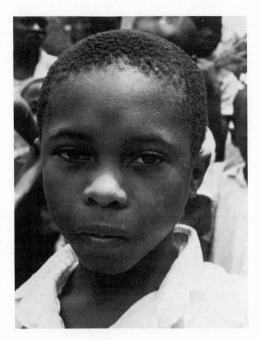

Figure 1.7. Onuchukwu Nwobodo, one of the *ogbanje* children.

concepts in Africa, it can be hard to pin down precise relationships, and the proof that I sought to establish a connection between the *ogbanje* and sickling has remained elusive. Nevertheless,
the link is highly suggestive and will be explored in Chapter 4.
But first we must turn to the remote past to try to reconstruct the
factors responsible for the origin of sickling cells and their impact
on African health and culture.

EVOLUTION AND HEMOGLOBIN

The qualities of *bricolage* that characterize certain aspects of both evolutionary processes in biology and cultural processes in traditional societies derive from a particular emphasis on the past. By contrast, highly industrialized, technological societies are oriented predominantly toward the future, with changes taking place so rapidly that we accept change as normal. However, in traditional African cultures, changes in customs and practices are usually so slow as to be virtually imperceptible. For the Igbo, it is impossible to identify a time before there were *ogbanjes*. Change is of course even slower on the time scale of evolution. The hemoglobin circulating in our blood is identical in every way to the hemoglobin that was in our ancestors a million years ago. Thus, in our quest to understand sickle cell anemia and its possible role in African society, we must turn to the past to begin to understand the present, both in cultural and biochemical terms.

The biochemical heritage of all living forms revolves around the four types of nucleotide bases that occur in DNA, the molecules of genetic inheritance, and the 20 types of amino acids that occur in proteins, the broad and versatile class of molecules responsible for most biochemical reactions. Deducing the exact relationship whereby a certain sequence of bases in the DNA of a gene specifies the amino acid sequence of the corresponding protein—that is, breaking the genetic code—was one of the great successes of molecular biology. Presumably, these bases and amino acids, as well as the building blocks for carbohydrates and fats, first formed spontaneously billions of years ago in the watery environment of early earth. Then, by some seemingly ineluctable but wholly mysterious processes, the first cells appeared and life was on its way.

The origins of hemoglobin go back hundreds of millions of years, to the first vertebrates that swam in the oceans of the planet. Although proteins clearly related to the hemoglobin of red blood cells have occurred sporadically among invertebrates, and even in certain plants, only with vertebrates is hemoglobin systematically encountered in the specialized red blood cells devoted to oxygen transport. These cells greatly increase the amount of oxygen that can be dissolved in the blood, thereby permitting the evolution of large bodies capable of rapid movements. First, a single type of hemoglobin chain existed, as still can be found in the blood of the lamprey eel. A related protein found in vertebrate muscle—myoglobin—also exists as a single chain. Then, in the period of divergence of lamprey from other vertebrate forms, a gene duplication occurred that led to two types of hemoglobin genes that produce different kinds of hemoglobin chains, known as alpha and beta. Two copies of each type associate together to give the typical hemoglobin molecule, with its four-part (tetrameric) structure.

Hemoglobin is found in a similar tetrameric form in fish, amphibia, reptiles, birds, and mammals. For most species, different tetrameric forms are found for different periods in the development of the organism. For example, in amphibia, the hemoglobin molecules in the tadpole differ from those in the adult. Humans progress from embryonic hemoglobin at the earliest stages of prenatal life, to fetal hemoglobin until birth, to the adult form that occurs throughout postnatal life. In the adult hemoglobin of humans, usually abbreviated as hemoglobin A, the alpha chains are made up of a sequence of 141 amino acids, while the beta chains contain 146 amino acids. Overall, the two types of chains are fairly similar, with the same amino acid occurring in about 50% of the corresponding positions of alpha and beta chains.

When hemoglobin molecules from many vertebrate species were studied in detail, differences in their amino acid sequences were observed that revealed two kinds of information. First, a limited number of positions were found to be invariant, that is, the

same type of amino acid was found at that position for every hemoglobin examined. The specific properties of the particular
amino acid were then considered to be essential at that position
and any changes in the course of evolution could not therefore be
tolerated. Second, at other positions (the vast majority), different
amino acids could be found in different species. Since in almost
all cases the differences did not appear to be correlated with any
significant change in the functional properties of hemoglobin, it
was assumed that the effects of the change were "neutral" and
simply reflect the accumulation of random mutations that occur
at a low frequency during DNA replication. Certain mutants may
have occurred that were highly deleterious, but presumably they
were eliminated by natural selection. Overall, the effect of random changes is to cause the hemoglobin sequences of species to
drift apart once they have diverged from a common ancestor. The
longer the time since the divergence, the greater the number of
differences that would be expected. Therefore, differences in hemoglobin sequence can serve as a valuable clock which measures
how long ago the species diverged from a common ancestor. Indeed, the concept of a biological clock in the genes was first applied by Emil Zuckerkandl and Linus Pauling in 1962 using data
from the hemoglobins of different species.[1]

It has been estimated that changes in the hemoglobin genes accumulate at the rate of 1 per alpha or beta chain every 2–3 million years.[2] This notion fits with our general ideas of evolution, as
we find 8 differences in the hemoglobin beta chains of humans
and rhesus monkeys, 24 differences between humans and cows, 45
differences between humans and chickens, and 91 differences between humans and sharks. Therefore, the longer the time since
any two species had a common ancestor, the greater the number
of differences that have accumulated. When the hemoglobins of
primates were compared, however, absolutely no difference in the
hemoglobin sequences of humans and chimpanzees could be
found. The similarity of these proteins suggested that chimpanzees and humans diverged from a common ancestor within the
last 2 million years, much more recently than had been previously
thought on the basis of fossil evidence.

Primate fossils had revealed progressive changes in features
(especially teeth, which are often the best preserved elements)
since primates first appeared some 70 million years ago. Thus, the

face of our primate ancestors changed on a time scale that coincided with changes in the face of the earth, as continents moved from their early locations within one extensive mass to their current positions. The first primate, a tiny creature about the size of a rat, was a contemporary of the dinosaurs and possessed 44 teeth (compared with 32 in adult humans). By 35 million years ago, a primate called *Aegyptopithecus* (ape from Egypt, because its fossil remains were discovered at Fayoum, Egypt) had evolved. About the size of a cat, it had the same number of teeth as humans, although its brain was still very small (27 cc). About this time the New World monkeys first appeared, with 36 teeth and a remarkable tail that functions almost like an extra hand. Perhaps the added advantages of this fifth appendage diminished the pressure for other changes, so that the eventual evolution of apes and humans was strictly an Old World phenomenon.[3]

Before the biochemical evidence indicated a more recent divergence of humans and apes, anthropologists had postulated that *Aegyptopithecus* was the last common ancestor of humans and apes. Now, however, we look to much more recent fossils and follow evolution from *Aegyptopithecus* to *Proconsul*, a species unearthed in Kenya, whose brain measured 150 cc. From *Proconsul*, we are led to *Dryopithecus* and *Kenyapithecus*, the latter appearing to be an especially promising link on the path to humans. *Kenyapithecus* existed after the collision of Africa (and Saudi Arabia) with Asia about 17 million years ago and may have given rise to *Ramapithecus*, the forerunner of the Asian apes, such as the orangutan. With its brain of 300 cc and late erupting molars (a sign of prolonged adolescence), *Kenyapithecus* has a number of features that suggest an ancestry for humans and apes. However, the time of the divergence of humans and apes from a common ancestor is still uncertain. The data from several biochemical measures suggest a time of 5–10 million years ago, although the results from hemoglobin alone would indicate a more recent divergence.

At the level of protein comparisons there are no differences between humans and chimpanzees not only in the adult form of their hemoglobin but also in several other proteins, and only minor differences suggested in the amino acid sequence, reaction with antibodies, and mobility in electrophoresis for other proteins. Even at the level of overall chromosome structure, there is striking similarity. Chimpanzees have one more pair of chromosomes than humans, but detailed structural studies show that one of the longer human chromosomes closely resembles a fused version of two of the shorter chimpanzee chromosomes. A schematic representation of the chromosomes of humans, chimpanzees, gorillas, and orangutans is presented in Figure 2.1. Like chimpanzees, gorillas and orangutans have 48 chromosomes, in contrast to the 46 chromosomes of humans. Chimpanzee chromosomes are generally regarded to be most similar to human chromosomes, and orangutan chromosomes least similar, although some experts have emphasized certain respects (such as the size of the Y chromosomes) in which gorilla chromosomes resemble human chromosomes even more closely than do chimpanzee chromosomes. Other experts have maintained that, chromosomes aside, by many anatomical criteria the orangutan is more closely related to humans than is either the chimpanzee or the gorilla.[4]

Another way to study the relatedness of humans to the other primates is to observe their behavior, since behavior is inherited along with chromosomes and proteins. The pioneering work of Jane Goodall in Tanzania reveals that chimpanzees possess certain aggressive traits, including the killing of members of their own species and acts of cannibalism, that were previously thought to be uniquely human qualities. Behavioral studies of gorillas in Rwanda by Dian Fossey reveal that gorilla males are more solitary creatures than chimpanzee males, which suggests to some researchers that they are less similar to humans than are chimpanzees. Unfortunately, the gorilla population in Central Africa may soon be extinct, if heroic measures are not taken soon to stop their wanton killing by poachers. Gorilla hands, for reasons impossible to comprehend, bring a high price for use as decorative ornaments and ashtrays.[5]

Thus, arguments from molecules to anatomy and behavior can be applied to questions about the relatedness of primates, and it is not easy to decide which arguments are the most important. However, certain facts lead to virtually inescapable conclusions, as is the case with data on hemoglobins from humans, chimpanzees, and gorillas. We have already noted that the hemoglobins of humans and chimpanzees are identical. Gorilla hemoglobin, however, does show one difference from human hemoglobin in each type of chain. In human and chimpanzee hemoglobin glutamic acid appears at position alpha 23 and arginine at position beta

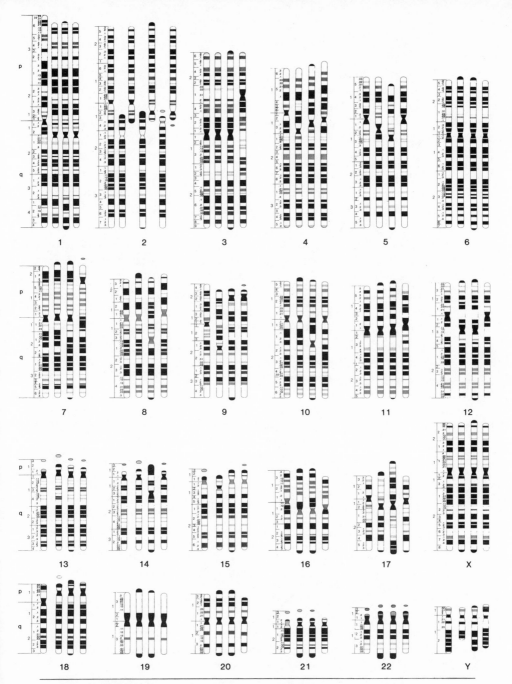

Figure 2.1. Schematic representation of the chromosomes of (from left to right) humans, chimpanzees, gorillas, and orangutans, arranged by chromosome size. The bands correspond to the locations of specific dye markings. (From Yunis and Prakas, 1982; copyright by the AAAS.)

104, whereas in gorilla hemoglobin aspartic acid and lysine, re-spectively, appear at these two positions. It is difficult to imagine any explanation for these facts other than a divergence from a common Homininae ancestor of two evolutionary lines, one lead-ing to gorillas and the other leading to humans and chimpanzees (Fig. 2.2).

In all probability, the change in the alpha chains (at position 23) occurred in the line to humans and chimpanzees, while the change in the beta chains (at position 104) occurred in the line to gorillas. This conclusion follows from the fact that orangutans, New World monkeys, and gibbons all share with gorillas an aspartic acid at position alpha 23. The evolutionary line leading to orangutans (Ponginae) must have diverged from the common Hominidae ancestor well before the split leading to gorillas versus humans and chimpanzees, since orangutans differ from the other three at two other locations in the beta chains (positions 87 and 125) and at position 12 in the alpha chains.[6] Thus, the difficulties in establishing degrees of relatedness for humans, chimpanzees, gorillas, and orangutans from chromosome patterns and features

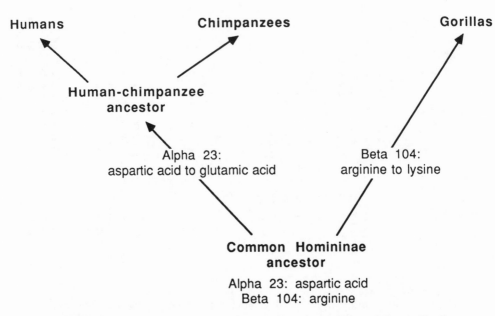

Figure 2.2. The divergence of the human–chimpanzee line and the gorilla line from a common Homininae ancestor.

of anatomy and behavior are resolved easily and in a straightfor-
ward manner by hemoglobin sequences. Any other interpretation
would have to invoke several extremely unlikely events. For example, if chimpanzees and gorillas had a common ancestor after
the split of the line to humans, we would need to postulate that by
coincidence, the line to humans and the line to chimpanzees
spontaneously, but separately, experienced the aspartic to glutamic change at position alpha 23. Alternatively, the change at
alpha 23 could have occurred in a common ancestor, but the line
to gorillas would have to have experienced a reversal of this
change, in addition to the change at beta 104. While these unlikely coincidences cannot be absolutely excluded, they have such
a small probability that they are effectively eliminated.

To dramatize the argument, we can formulate an analogy concerning a book with several editions. Imagine that Darwin's *Origin
of Species,* originally printed in Great Britain, was being reissued at
various times in English-language editions in several parts of the
world, say the United States, Australia, and Taiwan. Suppose
that in the edition typeset in the United States we came across a
typo in which the word "clean" was replaced by the word "clear."
Only a single letter change is involved, and since the new word is
not nonsense, it escaped the proofreaders. We also discovered that
in both the Australia and Taiwan editions, a sole different typo
was found, "glide" replaced by "slide." As in the case of the first
typo, this one also escaped the attention of proofreaders. Now the
question is, which texts were copied by which typesetters? Naturally, we would assume that the original British text was copied
once in the United States, with the change of "clean" to "clear"
introduced, and once again in either Australia or Taiwan, when
the change from "glide" to "slide" was introduced. This second
edition, along with its "glide/slide" error, was then copied by the
typesetter of the third edition (Fig. 2.3). We cannot dismiss absolutely the possibility that, for example, the Taiwan edition was
copied from the United States edition, with the coincidence of including the same "glide" to "slide" typo introduced in Australia,
plus the accidental reversal of the "clean" to "clear" typo, but
such a possibility would obviously be extremely unlikely, as
would a common ancestor for chimpanzees and gorillas after the
divergence of humans.

While the hemoglobin data indicate the probable order of the

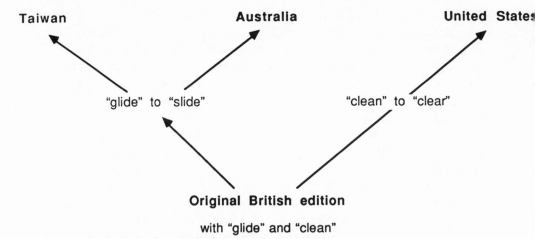

Figure 2.3. Hypothetical "divergence" of different editions of a book.

divergence of humans, chimpanzees, and gorillas, the time at which these divergences occurred is more difficult to estimate. The ticks of the biological clock that give rise to differences in genes are relatively infrequent. In addition, they are not regular, like a metronome, but represent only probabilities—a bit like waiting for earthquakes in California to measure the passage of time. A further complication is that the clock runs at different rates for different proteins, presumably slower if more portions of a protein are essential to its functions. When that is the case, changes are poorly tolerated and will tend to be excluded by evolution. The clock may also change its rate when major alterations in the protein occur, as appears to have been the case when evolution was leading to a hemoglobin with four subunits from ancestral forms with a single unit. If we calculate the time of the divergence of chimpanzee and human lines from their common ancestor on the basis of hemoglobin sequences, we would conclude that the divergence occurred only 1–2 million years ago. This recent a date would be impossible to reconcile with the generally accepted view (based on fossil evidence) that humans evolved from *Australopithecus* ancestors living in East Africa, whose remains go back 4–5 million years.

The discoveries of the various fossils now identified with *Australopithecus* began with Raymond Dart's description in 1925 of the Taung child skull from the Transvaal of South Africa. The claims of Dart were met initially with skepticism, and the eventual acceptance of *Australopithecus* was as much a credit to the perseverance of Dart and other early investigators as to the weight of the evidence. In the thinking of the time, Dart's discovery was surprising, since the expectations were for a big-brained creature with apelike teeth, just the opposite of Dart's small-brained being with humanlike teeth. Although the entire fossil record of *Australopithecus* could fit in a small suitcase, individual investigators have emphasized distinguishing features of their findings to justify naming a new species. Thus we have:

1. Dart's *Australopithecus africanus,* the original gracile type;

2. Robert Broom's *Australopithecus robustus,* a more heavy-boned form also found in South Africa (at Sterkfontein) in the period following Dart's discovery;

3. *Australopithecus boisei,* a form more solidly built than *robustus* that occurred in East Africa and was named for the Leakys' English sponsor, Charles Boise;

4. *Australopithecus afarensis,* the possible forerunner of the others, named by Donald Johanson, Timothy White, and Yves Coppens.

This last group includes the most intact remains of a single individual discovered to date; she was nicknamed Lucy by the discoverers (and called *birkinesh* by the Ethiopians, meaning "you are a person of value" in Amharic).[7]

The hind limbs of all the *Australopithecus* fossils indicate largely upright locomotion, and the heavy jaw structure indicates a mainly vegetarian diet. By the time of the australopithecines, the collision of the African continent with Asia had led to the formation of the great East African Rift Valley, with accompanying climatic changes that led to fewer trees and more open plains. According to arguments advanced especially by Coppens, primate ancestors isolated in East Africa may have then experienced strong selective pressure from the altered habitat to develop an upright posture for walking, in order to facilitate hunting and gathering in the open plains. In contrast, on the west side of the rift valley, the wetter conditions and lush vegetation favored development of gorillas and chimpanzees, which thrive in an arboreal habitat. Thus 4–5 million years ago, perhaps as a direct consequence of the earlier "tectonic accident," we would begin to find evidence of *Australopithecus* forms such as *afarensis*, with a brain size of about 500 cc, centered about what is currently Kenya (Fig. 2.4). This species was to be followed in the same region a million or so years later by *Homo habilis*, whose brain measured about 800 cc, roughly half the capacity of contemporary humans but well beyond the 400 cc of chimpanzees or 500 cc of gorillas.[8]

In addition to the line leading to *Homo*, the early australopithecines led to the later forms *boisei* in East Africa and *africanus* and *robustus* in South Africa. The various *Australopithecus* forms would become extinct at 1–1.5 million years ago. Thus, for a long period beginning some 2 million years ago, they lived side by side with *Homo habilis*, each surviving with some specialization: *Australopith-*

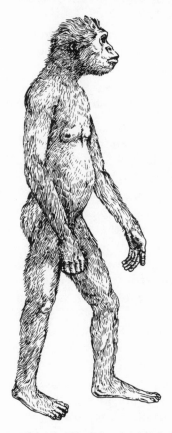

Figure 2.4. *Australopithecus afarensis.* (Drawing by Michel Garcia under the scientific direction of Yves Coppens.)

ecus was more developed as gatherers and *Homo habilis* as hunters. Thus, *Australopithecus* represents at different times both an ancestor and a cousin. Such patterns are common throughout evolution, where the divergence of two species yields one form that more closely resembles the common ancestor than does the other. The long cohabitation of *Australopithecus* "chewers" and *Homo habilis* "chasers" eventually ended with the disappearance of *Australopithecus* and the evolution of *Homo habilis* to a more mobile form, *Homo erectus*. It would seem that there was greater survival potential in the peripatetic life of the hunters compared with the gatherers.

Homo habilis had a more upright posture than *Australopithecus* and more humanlike teeth and jaws, indicating a more carnivorous diet. With its use of simple stone tools and its humanlike mouth, *Homo habilis* has much to identify it as nearly human, perhaps even language (see below). Then, about 1.5 million years ago, we find the appearance of *Homo erectus,* a species that occupied a large part of Africa, Europe, and Asia. The rise of *erectus* coincides with the passage from the simple stone tools of the pebble culture to the Acheulean industry with its long-enduring "biface" tool (Fig. 2.5). This tool, created by a characteristic striking of one stone with another, was to last as the principal invention of *Homo* for nearly a million years. *Homo erectus* also domesticated fire, specialized his shelters, and perhaps performed rituals related to death, since many skulls several hundreds of thousands of years old appear to be deliberately broken in a similar way, as if to remove the brain or destroy the face. It was with the appearance of *Homo sapiens neanderthalis* in the last 100,000 years and then the appearance of *Homo sapiens sapiens* some 40,000 years ago that our species was achieved. Although *neanderthalis* is an unpopular ancestor—no one appears to relish descent from what has been characterized as a brutish-looking creature, these individuals had an advanced culture of stone tools, cave art, and ritual burials that is similar to that of such groups as Cro-Magnon, which have been identified as *Homo sapiens sapiens*. Most likely, *Homo sapiens neanderthalis* is not an ancestor of modern humans but a relatively short-lived cousin.

While this scenario of human ancestry via *Australopithecus*-like ancestors is generally accepted by current anthropologists, it would place the human–chimpanzee divergence at least 5 million

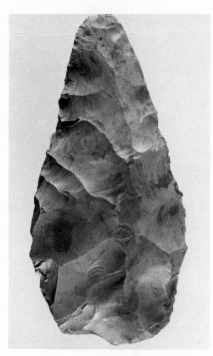

Figure 2.5. The biface, a tool typical of the industries of the Stone Age. (From Musée de l'Homme, Paris. Photographed by M. Delaplanche.) Length: 177mm.

years ago. However, if this estimate is correct, why are chimpanzee and human hemoglobins identical, suggesting a divergence only 1–2 million years ago? Most likely, the identical hemoglobins can be explained by the random striking of the biological clock. Since the biological clock measured by amino acid replacements is only a statistical probability, fluctations in rate are always occurring. Therefore, we can postulate that this biological clock just happened not to tick during the period since they last shared an ancestor. This is the simplest argument to reconcile the various lines of evidence. Since only one or two ticks would have been expected, no ticks is not a very different outcome. If we were to watch an hourglass with sensitive instruments that indicate one grain of sand passing on the average every millisecond, it would not be too surprising to find one or two milliseconds going by occasionally with no grains of sand falling. Nevertheless, scientists are often uncomfortable leaving explanations to such whims of chance; consequently, other possibilities have been proposed.

One hypothesis favored by Morris Goodman to explain the apparent incompatibility of the hemoglobin sequences with the fossil evidence is that the hemoglobin biological clock slowed down. In this argument, the rate of evolution slowed specifically during late primate evolution owing to a perfection of the hemoglobin molecules; selection mechanisms simply would not tolerate any further changes. I find this argument very hard to accept, since the function of hemoglobin in humans and chimpanzees is not noticeably changed from that in other primates whose hemoglobin structure is nevertheless different; a structure like hemoglobin can easily tolerate changes on the surface without any deleterious consequences. For nine globins from distant species that have been studied in full three-dimensional detail by x-ray crystallography, the basic structure is retained even though the amino acid sequences are only 17% the same for the most different globins.[9] In the evolution of proteins, there will always be a steady flux of changes, as an amino acid replacement in one region of the molecule compensates for a change in a nearby amino acid. Proteins are dynamic structures and many different combinations of amino acid sequence may achieve comparable success in carrying out the functions of the protein. Therefore, it is difficult to credit the idea that evolution of hemoglobin has suddenly achieved perfection in the human and chimpanzee lines in a way that would not tolerate any amino acid replacements.

In summary, we can conclude quite safely that hemoglobin is not a precise biological clock for relatively short times. Nevertheless, the fossil evidence should also be scrutinized for alternative explanations. We might imagine that *Australopithecus,* or even *Homo habilis,* was not on the line to humans but rather represents an evolutionary blind alley; the humanlike features might be due to parallel or even convergent evolution. Our understanding of the late stages of primate evolution is further complicated by recent revisions in general concepts of evolution. In the past, evolutionists have tended to view the development of species in terms of gradual but steady changes that take place in imperceptibly small increments. In the current thinking on evolution, typified by the writings of Stephen Jay Gould, there has been a shift away from the idea of gradual changes in favor of more punctuated processes.[10] In this view, species are relatively stable for long periods. Then dramatic mutational events, perhaps coinciding with

major environmental changes, trigger a brief period of rapid evolution in populations which eventually settle down, leaving new
species that remain relatively stable. The fossil records of many
species are consistent with the punctuated process: numerous
groups of species appear unchanged over long periods of the geological record, only to undergo apparently rapid evolution over a
short period of time.

The late stages of human evolution provide an example of a period of rapid change. In such periods, many different potential
lines of evolution may be launched, with only a small number ultimately succeeding to produce enduring species. Thus, arguing
from the fossil record is always problematic, especially during periods of rapid change. A few powerful genetic changes have led to
the greatly increased brain size and the accompanying behavioral
differences between humans and chimpanzees. Conceivably, the
circumstances that precipitated these events could have occurred
more than once, with the events that actually led to humans taking place more recently than the time of *Australopithecus*. We know
from the evolution of other species that such parallel evolution is
possible. For example, a now-extinct horse-like form known as
Thoatherium arose in South America in a line of evolution that was
independent of the modern horse.[11]

If the genes that have been studied so far are an accurate reflection of the two species' genomes, the genetic differences between humans and chimpanzees are extremely subtle. In some
cases possibly merely the timing of the activation of certain genes
has been altered so as to elongate the early development of
humans. It has been noted, for example, that there is a marked
similarity in skull structure in juvenile chimpanzees and adult
humans (Fig. 2.6). Therefore, it could be argued that the seemingly limitless capacity of humans to learn and adapt at all stages
of life reflects certain developmental processes in which the entire
human life span is an expanded and enriched version of chimpanzee childhood. Once such a developmental change was initiated in evolution, it could have reached its full application
relatively quickly, particularly in association with the evolution of
social behavior that permitted longer periods of childhood de-
pendency. In this way, the social component of evolution could
have permitted an accelerated evolutionary process compatible

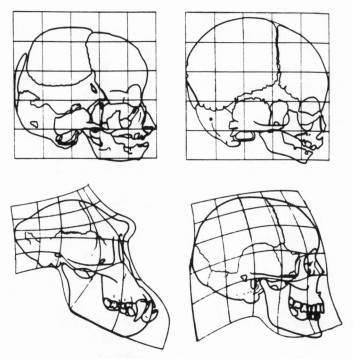

Figure. 2.6. Features of skulls from juvenile (upper two) and adult (lower two) chimpanzees (on the left) and humans (on the right). (From Starck and Kummer, 1962.)

with the divergence of humans and chimpanzees from their common ancestor even as recently as 1–2 million years ago.

The transition from 48 chromosomes in the human–chimpanzee ancestor to 46 chromosomes in humans would act as a partial sterility barrier between humans and the ancestral line, and this partial genetic isolation would have accelerated the development of human traits. Individuals that inherit 24 chromosomes from one parent and 23 from the other would not have correct pairing of the chromosomes, and as a result meiosis (formation of eggs or sperm) would be defective about half the time. Therefore, "hybrid" individuals with 47 chromosomes would be strongly selected against. As we noted earlier, the reduction in chromosome number for humans probably arose from a fusion of two chromosomes found in chimpanzees and other primates. We can safely assume that this event occurred only once, to give an individual with 47 chromosomes. Upon mating with an individual with 48 chromosomes, the number of their offspring would be limited by the partial sterility barrier, but half would have 47 chromosomes. Then possibly incest played a role, as implied in the biblical legend of Genesis, with the male and female offspring of two 47-chromosome parents inheriting 46 chromosomes and starting the human race. Were the 46-chromosome individuals to have arisen after the appearance of *Australopithecus,* these fascinating creatures may have been only an evolutionary cul de sac, and not on the line to humans.

The question of when humans and chimpanzees diverged is not likely to be settled conclusively until a great deal more information is available, both about the biochemical differences between the two species and about the fossil record. Nevertheless, a split of the human and chimpanzee lines about 5–6 million years ago (a figure compatible with the assumption that early *Australopithecus* was a human ancestor) appears to be increasingly likely on the basis of data from a number of sources. For example, recent analyses of regions of DNA that are in the vicinity of the beta globin genes but do not code for proteins are consistent with a divergence between chimpanzees and humans some 6 million years ago. Other results, including the overall similarity of human and chimpanzee DNA and the difference of one amino acid in their myoglobins, also support a divergence in this period.[12]

Regardless of the exact date of their divergence from a common ancestor, it is clear that humans and chimpanzees are extremely similar by biological standards. Indeed, according to generally accepted criteria of taxonomy applied throughout the animal kingdom, humans, chimpanzees, and gorillas should be members of the same genus, leading one observer to suggest that their designations might be recast by future primatologists as *Homo sapiens, Homo troglodytes* (derived from the current classification of chimpanzees as *Pan troglodytes*), and *Homo gorilla.*[13] Nevertheless, human beings sense that chimpanzees are worlds apart in certain essential respects, particularly in terms of language skills which distinguish humans so dramatically from their primate relatives.

One of the early successes of neurology was to link certain disorders in language skills, known categorically as aphasia, to damage at particular locations in the brain. More than 100 years ago, two of the founders of neurology, Paul Broca and then Carl Wernicke, described the linguistic differences between aphasias resulting from damage to different anatomical regions in the left hemisphere.

> The aphasic of the Broca's type characteristically produces little speech, which is emitted slowly, with great effort, and with poor articulation . . . the small grammatical words and endings are omitted. These patients show a surprising capacity to find single words. Thus, asked about the weather, the patient might say "Overcast." Urged to produce a sentence he may say, "Weather . . . overcast." These patients invariably show a comparable disorder in their written output, but they may comprehend spoken and written language normally. In striking contrast to these performances, the patient may retain his musical capacities. It is a common but most dramatic finding to observe a patient who produces single substantive words with great effort and poor articulation and yet sings a melody correctly and even elegantly.
>
> The Wernicke's asphasic contrasts sharply with the Broca's type. The speech output can be rapid and effortless, and in many cases the rate of production of words exceeds the normal. The output has the rhythm and melody of normal speech, but it is remarkably empty and conveys little or no information. The patient uses many filler words, and the speech is filled with circumlocutions. A typical production might be "I was over in the other one, and then after they had been in the department, I was in this one." The Wernicke's aphasic may, in writing, produce well-formed letters, but the output exhibits the same linguistic defects which are observed in the patient's speech.[14]

The specialization of the brain for language is further illustrated by the description of Japanese patients with aphasias of the Broca or Wernicke type who in some cases retain the ability to read and write *kanji,* the Chinese-derived characters. The recognition of these characters is apparently associated with the right hemisphere, which is the seat of image memory.

Fossil remains of *Homo habilis* show an enlargement of the region of the brain that Broca identified as a center of speech. Thus, to simple tools and varied diet, we should add perhaps language. While many think of *Homo erectus* or even *Homo sapiens* as the first species with language, for Yves Coppens,

> a long preoccupation with *Homo habilis* leads me to think, however, that it is likely to be to this species that questions should be ad-

dressed in order to know who we were, where we come from, and where we have been. Their sudden triumph under new conditions, wisely eating from varied sources, building huts, constructing tools with diverse forms reflecting diversified activities—I find these things so brilliant, so extraordinary, and so novel that I would readily choose this species, in its time and setting, to locate the appearance of consciousness and of language. We can say roughly speaking that these first men and women appeared as higher primates of the arid savana, walking erect, opportunists in their diets, conscious, and talkative. What has come to be called Man, in all his functional and behavioral characteristics, is there.[15]

A reconstitution of *Homo habilis* is presented in Figure 2.7.

These processes, initiated perhaps by *Homo habilis*, were perfected with the various *Homo* forms, leading to our *sapiens sapiens*.

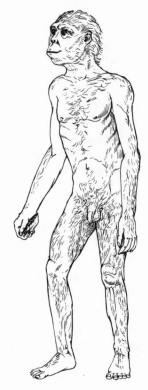

Figure 2.7. *Homo habilis*, the earliest *Homo* known. (Drawing by Michel Garcia under the scientific direction of Yves Coppens.)

Hunting and gathering gradually gave way to sedentary farming, and with the appearance of farm communities, relatively high population densities could be achieved. In Africa, these conditions led eventually to the spread of malaria and the selection of sickle hemoglobin. We have seen how hemoglobin changes can be used as a tool to distinguish between alternative views of primate evolution, but under conditions where hemoglobins varied little, if at all, during millions of years. Now we must explore the circumstances that led to the evolution of a hemoglobin variant responsible for sickling on a reduced scale of "microevolution," involving probably only a few thousand years.

THE MICROEVOLUTION OF SICKLING

In contrast with the dramatic steps in the evolution of humans from their primate ancestors, the events that led to sickling represent a more limited process, yet one that changed hemoglobin molecules for the first time in some 5 million years, as far as we can judge, for a significant fraction of the human population in Africa. We shall now try to discover how hemoglobin that had remained constant for so long could appear in an altered form in millions of people in a relatively short period of time.

The critical events in the rise of the sickle mutation almost certainly occurred during recorded history—a time scale in which centuries once again assume importance. To bring us back to this perspective, we only need note that it was just somewhat more than a century ago (1864) that a German scientist, Felix Hoppe-Seyler, named the red substance from blood "hemoglobin." Observations with the earliest microscopes had established in the 1600s that the red color of blood was packaged in multitudes of tiny cells or "globules." The name hemoglobin reflects the source of the material from globules (hence "globin") and from blood (hence the prefix "hemo-" from the Greek word *haima*, meaning "blood").[1] Hoppe-Seyler's laboratory in Tübingen achieved renown for these studies of hemoglobin and also as the setting for the first isolation of DNA by his colleague Frederich Miescher. In contrast, another scientist working at this time in what is now

Czechoslovakia went largely unnoticed. His name was Gregor Mendel.

Mendel, an Augustinian monk, performed as a sideline to his monastic duties extraordinary experiments that laid the foundation of modern genetics. His findings were published by the Brno Society of Natural Science in 1865 in a paper entitled "Experiments on Plant Hybrids." However, the *Journal of the Brno Society* was not in the mainstream of scientific publications. Although 120 libraries received copies of the journal, the significance of Mendel's article was not appreciated in scientific circles until it was rediscovered at the turn of the century. Once his findings were thoroughly exposed to the scientific community, Mendel was recognized as an exceptionally gifted scientist. Unfortunately, the recognition came too late to provide satisfaction to Mendel, who died in 1884.

Mendel carried out his experiments with the common garden pea. He worked with different strains that possessed well-defined characteristics: some plants produced round peas and others produced wrinkled peas. He noticed that in his many crosses between the plants with round peas and those with wrinkled peas, the first generation hybrid always produced round peas. The following year, Mendel would cross many of these first generation hybrid plants. In this way, he obtained 7,324 second generation peas, of which 5,474 were round and 1,850 were wrinkled. The ratio of round to wrinkled was 2.96:1, or (within experimental error) 3:1. Experiments of this type were repeated with plants having other readily observable characteristics. In every case of two alternative parental characters, only one appeared in the first generation hybrids. Moreover, the character that vanished in the first generation hybrids always reappeared among one-fourth of the population of the crosses between the hybrids.

On the basis of these observations, Mendel reasoned that the characters responsible for the heredity of the form of the pea are carried and passed on to the next generation in discrete units. Each pea must possess a pair of such units, with one of the two producing the dominant characteristic, such as round peas (abbreviated R), and the other producing the recessive characteristic, such as wrinkled peas (abbreviated W). In the hybrids, both are present, but only the character of the dominant unit is expressed.

When two hybrids are crossed, four kinds of peas will be produced in statistically equal amounts, based on the alternative combinations of the individual heredity characters.

Cross: Hybrid 1   ×   Hybrid 2
              R_1/W_1 R_2/W_2

Peas: R_1/R_2 R_1/W_2 W_1/R_2 W_1/W_2

The wrinkled exterior of the recessive unit of heredity manifests itself in only the one-fourth of the population that is homozygous for W, the W_1/W_2 group. The other three-fourths would appear round, although they would be actually a mixture of homozygous forms (R_1/R_2) and heterozygous forms (R_1/W_2 and W_1/R_2).

The two types of wrinkled peas reveal that it is possible to distinguish between the composition of the genes, called "genotype," and the physical appearance of the living organism, called "phenotype." For the homozygous R_1/R_2 and W_1/W_2 plants, the genotype corresponds exactly to the phenotype. However, for the hybrid R_1/W_2 or W_1/R_2 plants, the phenotype appears the same as R_1/R_2 plants, although the genotype is heterozygous for the R and W genes. Thus, an important aspect of Mendel's insights was distinguishing between the genotype and phenotype. The brilliance of Mendel's deductions shines all the more brightly when compared with the impoverished ideas on the subject of inheritance advanced in the same period by Darwin. As noted by Stent and Calendar, "Indeed, Darwin's 'pangenesis' concept of the mechanism of heredity, which envisages that each part of the adult organism produces 'gemmules' which are collected in the 'seed' for transmission to the offspring, was more or less the same as that propounded by Hippocrates some twenty-three centuries earlier."[2]

Although formulated with peas, the principles Mendel discovered apply to the genes for hemoglobin and its sickle variant. When the mutant form of hemoglobin associated with sickling cells was first detected in 1949 by Linus Pauling and his colleagues, they gave it the designation "hemoglobin S" ("S" for "sickle"). The individuals who are heterozygous for the sickle mutation, that is, the carriers of sickle trait, can be designated as "hybrids," since they possess genes for both hemoglobin A and hemoglobin S. The children of two such hybrids (or carriers) will

receive the chromosomes from each parent according to four possibilities of equal probability. The four possibilities are analogous
to the four categories of genes for round and wrinkled peas. If we
designate the genes of the father by adding f and those of the
mother by adding m, the hemoglobin A and S genes will be dis-
tributed as follows:

Parents: Father   ×   Mother
                    A_f/S_f A_m/S_m

Children: A_f/A_m A_f/S_m A_m/S_f S_f/S_m

The sickle character is essentially "recessive," since cells carrying an S gene do not normally sickle if the A gene is also present.
On the average, the recessive character of sickled cells will be fully
manifested in only the 25% of the children who possess the S_f/S_m
genes. These children will have sickle cell anemia. The normal hemoglobin gene will be expressed in the other 75% of the children,
who would be a mixture of individuals with only normal hemoglobin (A_f/A_m) and hybrid individuals with both hemoglobins
(A_f/S_m and A_m/S_f). These latter individuals, while appearing
normal because of the dominance of the A gene over the S, are
carriers of sickle trait who can pass the gene on to their children.
If two such second-generation carriers marry, the risk is again 1 in
4 that their children will have sickle cell anemia.[3]

We can abbreviate the scheme depicted above by denoting hemoglobin genes as simply A or S. Individuals can then be identified by their genotype and designated simply as AA, AS, and SS.
According to the Mendelian scheme, then, for children of two
carriers, the probability of the ratios of offspring are AA:AS:SS =
1:2:1.

If the sickle mutation had arisen only once and had followed
the 1:2:1 ratio with no additional factors, we would not be discussing it now, since it would never have reached the proportions that
make it a major medical problem among individuals of African
descent. However, the fact that the sickle mutation appears to
have increased the resistance of AS individuals to malaria has led
to the proliferation of carriers in the mosquito-infested African
tropics. The eventual consequence has been that African children
in increasing numbers have had two AS individuals as parents,
and the unlucky 1 in 4 of these children has developed sickle cell

anemia. Any benefits these SS children might have in fighting malaria are heavily outweighed by the many deleterious consequences of sickling cells.

We can now formulate more quantitatively how the sickle mutation came to such abundance in Africa. We must assume that the AS individuals had some advantage over both AA individuals and SS individuals. The reproductive fitness of the SS individuals would have been diminished by the health problems associated with having sickling cells. The AA individuals would have been plagued somewhat more than AS individuals by the effects of malaria. It appears that the advantage of AS individuals over AA individuals in resisting malaria occurs especially in the early childhood years before children develop a degree of acquired immunity from their own antibody production. This view is consistent with the finding in Nigeria that fatal cases of malaria are almost invariably in infants, but precise estimates on the relative fitness of AA, AS, and SS individuals are difficult to obtain.[4] Only limited data exists for the relative advantages of AS over AA individuals in resisting malaria; and, as we shall see, different studies have yielded conflicting results. Laboratory studies on the growth of the malaria parasite *Plasmodium falciparum* in red cells from AA, AS, and SS individuals have helped to reveal the molecular mechanism of the protection for AS individuals (see Chapter 6). However, studies at the cellular level do not provide information on the reproductive fitness of the individuals with these cells. Nevertheless, the weight of the evidence indicates that, in all probability, the effect of one S gene is relatively small; only on the order of 10% more AS than AA individuals survive to reproduce in every generation. The fitness handicap of SS individuals is also difficult to estimate, especially for historical times in Africa. Data from contemporary medical clinics and information available from field studies suggest that the presence of two S genes often has a devastating effect on Africans. The majority of these homozygous individuals succumb before becoming parents; and SS females who do survive to reproductive maturity are rarely able to surmount the strains of pregnancy.

The fragility and shortened life time of sickling red blood cells causes a state of weakness associated with anemia in general. However, the anemia per se is a relatively minor aspect of the overall problems associated with sickling cells. In fact, these other problems would probably be aggravated were the anemia lessened, since sickled cells cause blockages of circulation and more cells would worsen the obstructions. Other than the anemia associated with sickling cells, there are three severe types of problems faced by SS individuals: (1) greatly heightened susceptibility to bacterial infection, particularly in the early childhood years; (2) painful episodes (vaso-occlusive crises) associated with blockages in the circulatory system; and (3) progressive degeneration of various organs of the body caused by impaired circulation.[5]

Concerning the risks to life in the early years, it has been shown that evidence of cell sickling can be found as early as 3 months. Prior to that age, the red cells contain appreciable amounts of the fetal form of hemoglobin which provide some protection against sickling. Once hemoglobin S predominates, high risks are encountered. From studies conducted in the United States we know that infants with sickle cell anemia have died suddenly due to infections, particularly pneumoccocal sepsis and meningitis and to a lesser degree salmonella, shigella, and tuberculosis. Corresponding studies in Ghana indicate similar susceptibility to infections, although commonly with malaria and typhoid.[6] The incidence of malaria infection indicates that in spite of whatever resistance to malaria AS individuals may have, young SS individuals suffer from an overall susceptibility to infection that overwhelms any slight resistance to malaria that might have been associated directly with the S gene.

The childhood infections of SS infants arise mainly from loss of the functions of the spleen. Its extensive capillaries are among the first to be blocked by sickled cells; the result is usually a small, nonfunctional spleen by mid-childhood. Evidence of impaired spleen function can generally be detected in SS infants less than one year old. Progressive diminution in size of the spleen occurs, with SS children generally functionally asplenic by the age of 7. Since the spleen plays a role in the defenses of the body to infection, particularly from bacterial sources, homozygous SS children become acutely susceptible to infection. Overturf and Powers site data indicating an incidence of bacterial meningitis 25 times higher in children with sickle cell anemia than in normal children; the incidence of salmonellosis was found to be some 300 times higher. In a number of clinical centers, regular administration of prophylactic antibiotics has led to a marked improvement in the health and survival of the population treated. Pneumococcal vaccines have also been used with modest success.

It is now clear that young children carefully monitored and promptly treated at the first signs of infection will have a good chance of surviving this critical period. Of course, such care was out of the question in Africa historically, and a large part of the mortality associated with sickle cell anemia was undoubtedly due to early childhood infections. While intense health-care practices to carry SS children through the early critical years are still relatively rare in Africa outside certain clinical centers in large cities, such practices are expected to become more widespread, and the population of adolescent and adult sicklers will continue to rise. As a result, the other consequences of the disease will become medical problems on an increasingly wide scale and will add to the sense of urgency to find a treatment for sickle cell anemia. These more long-term consequences are responsible for significant further mortality in those SS individuals who reach adolescence.

In general, the children with sickle cell anemia who approach adolescence experience slower growth than their normal peers; a delay of several years in the arrival of puberty is commonly encountered. However, delayed puberty leads to a continuation of growth beyond the usual age range, so that the final height of SS individuals is on the average within the normal range. Serious consequences may then arise from problems of circulation. In virtually all cases, impaired circulation leads to episodes of intense pain which begin suddenly and may last for days. The chest is one of the frequent points of pain, along with the abdomen or joints of the arms or legs. When these painful crises occur in young children, the hands and feet are common targets. Depending on the individual, crises may recur frequently (at intervals of a few weeks) or, for the fortunate few, only rarely, if at all. Treatment at the present time is limited to sedation, analgesics, and fluids.

Apart from these intense episodes of pain, there are a series of inevitable changes that take their toll as well. The lungs are subject to progressive damage, which leads to poor oxygenation of sickled red cells that already have difficulty in binding oxygen (see Chapter 6). Decreased oxygenation of the blood places stress on the heart, which tries to compensate for the low oxygen supply by pumping more blood. As a result, enlarged, hyperactive hearts are found in SS individuals. Liver and kidney damage is also encountered. Various signs of circulatory problems can be readily detected in the eyes of SS individuals as they age; sometimes the result is a loss of vision in adults. Skin ulcers, often around the ankles, are one of the most aggravating problems for SS individuals. In Africa, scars from healed leg ulcers are one of the signs used for preliminary diagnosis of a homozygous SS individual awaiting hemoglobin testing. Bone deformities are also encountered, either as a result of infections or as a general symptom, such as the biconcave shape of vertebra (described pictorially as "fishmouth" vertebra) typical of SS individuals. Indeed, one of the rare SS individuals I met in Africa outside of big city clinics was a teenage boy in the village of Awgu, where I first encountered the *ogbanje* children. When I asked how he had been diagnosed, he showed me the x-ray that he had proudly saved which revealed the typical deformation of the vertebra. In certain clinics an x-ray is more readily obtained than a hemoglobin analysis. I eventually obtained a blood sample from this boy and found that he was indeed homozygous SS.

On the basis of the information we have about the health problems encountered by SS individuals, as well as information from other sources, we can now pursue the issue of the fitness of AA, AS, and SS individuals in the African tropics. In order to develop quantitative arguments concerning the evolution of the sickle mutation, we must define the "fractional reproductive fitness"—the fractions of the population of AA, AS, and SS individuals that live at least long enough to reproduce. If we assign the AS individuals an arbitrary fitness of one, then the fitness for AA individuals is less than one, owing to their somewhat greater susceptibility to malaria, and the fitness of SS individuals is substantially less than one because of the problems caused by sickling:

Genotype	AA	AS	SS
Fitness	Fitness < 1	Fitness = 1	Fitness << 1

Since populations in Africa rarely exceed an incidence of AS individuals of about 30%, we can start our calculations by assuming that this is generally as high as the value can go. In other words, it has reached equilibrium. The final population of individuals with the sickle gene will thus be balanced by the advantages of malaria resistance versus the disadvantages of sickling. Relatively more AS individuals will be found when the AA mortality is specifically increased by a malaria environment. However, a high SS mortality will tend to limit the percentage of AS individuals by reducing the number of S genes in the population. These factors can be expressed mathematically using the equations of populations genetics for what is called a "balanced polymorphism."[7] The incidence of the S gene found in the Igbo population (and other comparable groups) is compatible with only a limited range of values for the relative reproductive fitness of AA individuals, even when the fitness of SS individuals varies widely, as summarized in Table 3.1.

Case 1 represents the lowest possible fitness for SS (zero), which corresponds to the possibility that SS individuals never reproduce. Under these circumstances a Fitness(AA) = 0.81 would be required to achieve the percentage typical of the Igbo of 25% AS. Therefore, 0.81 is the lower limit of Fitness(AA), since Fitness(SS) is certainly greater than zero and higher values of Fitness(SS) lead to higher estimates of Fitness(AA). As a result, Fitness(AA) must fall within the range 0.80–1.0, but a Fitness(AA) as high as 0.95 (Case 5) would require a Fitness(SS) = 0.74, which is unrealistically high. Comparison of Case 1 and Case 5 illustrates that the higher the Fitness(SS), the smaller the difference between Fitness(AA) and Fitness(AS) required to achieve 25% AS for the population. It is only when the Fitness(SS) is extremely poor, approaching zero, that the Fitness(AA) must be some 20% lower than Fitness(AS) in order to favor AS individuals to a degree sufficient to overcome the loss of S genes in the SS group.

Since Case 1 and Case 5 provide unlikely extremes, more

Table 3.1. Fitness values. Calculations are based on the following percentages at birth: AA = 73.4%; AS = 25%; SS = 1.6%.

| Case | Fitness | | |
	AA	AS	SS
1	0.81	1.0	0.00
2	0.83	1.0	0.10
3	0.85	1.0	0.22
4	0.90	1.0	0.48
5	0.95	1.0	0.74

plausible parameters are presented in Case 2 with Fitness(AA) = 0.83 and Fitness(SS) = 0.10, Case 3 with Fitness(AA) = 0.85 and Fitness(SS) = 0.22, and Case 4 with Fitness(AA) = 0.90 and Fitness(SS) = 0.48. Although there is insufficient evidence to distinguish with certainty which of these three cases best represents the past circumstances of the Igbo, the situation historically was probably closer to Case 2 or Case 3, since Fitness(SS) approaching 0.50 is difficult to reconcile with the multiple consequences of SS red cells. Therefore, we can tentatively conclude that for many generations in the African tropics, only about 9 AA individuals on the average for every 10 AS individuals survived to reproduce. At the same time, the SS individuals were plagued by the various childhood risks and the difficulties of adolescence, with young women in particular likely to succumb during the added stress of pregnancy, thereby contributing to an overall fitness of SS individuals of 0.10–0.50.

Since many African peoples have incidences of AS individuals that are far lower than 25%, we can assume either that for these people equilibrium has not yet been reached, or that if it has, then the relative advantages of the AS individuals are reduced. It is probably the latter case for certain populations, since the reduced incidence of AS generally coincides with drier climates which tend to be less supportive of the *Anopheles* mosquito that transmits the malaria parasite. As a result, malaria is probably less severe a problem in these areas and AA individuals are at less of a disadvantage compared with AS individuals than in wetter climates which support *Anopheles* growth. Diet may also be a factor (see below). Thus, the fitness of AA individuals (compared with AS at 1.0) may be considerably higher than 0.90 for population groups with a lower incidence of the S gene. The impression may have been created that AS individuals are almost always protected against malaria, but the mathematical arguments make it clear that the protection is only slight. Even in the critical childhood period, the protection of AS individuals from malaria is not readily measurable, as emphasized recently, for example, by Linda Jackson on the basis of her field work in Liberia.

This current view of only limited protection against malaria contrasts with early reports from A. C. Allison of a spectacular protection against malaria in AS individuals. When volunteers from the Luo ethnic group of East Africa were innoculated with malaria parasites, Allison reported in 1954 that 14 of 15 AA individuals developed malaria, compared with only 2 of 15 AS individuals. Ethical considerations aside, the relatively small number of individuals involved in this study and other questions of procedure make it difficult to draw firm conclusions from these results. Overall, the protection against malaria in AS individuals now is accepted to be much more modest.[8]

For our purposes, a principal reason for deducing a value of Fitness(AA) was to permit calculation of the microevolutionary time required for the S gene to reach its current incidence. Accepting the estimate of Fitness(AA) = 0.90, we can go on to the next step and consider the period of time during which the sickle gene was selected. We will then reconsider how sensitive the time period calculated is to the actual value for Fitness(AA).

In order to estimate the span of time required to account for the incidence of the sickle gene, we must make calculations that are similar to compounding interest on a bank account. As a first approximation, the value of Fitness(AA) = 0.90 means that AS individuals increased by roughly 10% in each generation until equilibrium was reached. We can ask how long it would have taken the AS individuals to double their share of the population. If money is placed in a bank account at 10% interest, it doubles in about 7 years. Similarly, the proportion of AS individuals would have doubled roughly every 7 generations. However, the estimates of the total time required to achieve current levels of the S gene are complicated by another factor, the size of the population affected.

Population groups which currently possess the sickle mutation to a significant degree comprise hundreds of millions of people. Nevertheless, if the sickle gene is at equilibrium, we can assume that it has been at equilibrium for some time, long enough that at an earlier time in history the affected group had a much smaller total population, say 10 million, and then grew with the same equilibrium values. If the sickle gene arose only once, within that population, it must have started at a time when the population was much smaller still, say 1 million.[9] Starting at a value of one AS individual in a group with a population of 1 million, we may ask how many times the percentage must double to reach a value of 25% AS in the population. If you could persuade someone to give you one penny on the first day of the month, two pennies on the second, four pennies on the third, eight pennies on the fourth, and so on, doubling the number of pennies every day to the end of the month, you would receive a billion pennies on the thirtieth day of the month. Clearly, doubling has a way of sneaking up on us. For our hypothetical case of the rise of AS individuals, to progress from one in a million to 25% of the population would take 17 doublings.

By various calculations, we have now assembled all the information necessary to estimate the time of hemoglobin S microevolution. If the incidence of AS individuals doubled every 7 generations and 17 doublings would bring us to current levels, we have a total of $7 \times 17 = 119$ generations. At about 20 years per generation, our estimate is that the evolution of sickling has been going on some 24 centuries, or 2,400 years. For many reasons, this is a rough estimate and could be off by many centuries. If SS individuals had even poorer reproductive fitness, which may well have been the case, with a value of Fitness(SS) approaching 0.20 or less, then Fitness(AA) would be reduced to 0.85 and the time estimates for the rise of AS individuals could be cut by hundreds of years. Since African women traditionally marry soon after puberty, the generation time may have been several years less than 20 years. Furthermore, we have neglected effects of migrations, which are known to have been major factors in African history.[10]

Migrations almost certainly played a role in the spread of the sickle gene, especially through central and southern Africa. While the diversity of languages in West Africa suggests independent origins for these languages several thousands of years ago, the Bantu languages of central and southern Africa are more closely related. Historical evidence indicates that this distribution reflects migrations of peoples who originated in the Benue River region in eastern Nigeria, where related languages are still spoken. The migrations are believed to have occurred in the first millennium B.C. and thus in the time period estimated for the origin of the sickle mutation. For reasons to be presented in Chapter 7, it would appear that the sickle gene arose independently among the Bantu peoples at an early stage of their migrations. Other migrations from the region of Nigeria toward the west are likely also to have contributed to the spread of the sickle gene.

Multiple origins of the sickle gene and migrations would change our estimates of population sizes somewhat, and would decrease our estimates of the time during which microevolution occurred. In contrast, when population densities were lower, malaria may have been less prevalent and the selective advantage of AS individuals compared with AA individuals would have been lower. Thus, there are a number of competing factors that are difficult to analyze, but the general trend of the calculations is probably valid, indicating origins for the sickle mutation in the time span of the first millennium B.C. to the first millennium A.D.

The influence of migrations of entire populations on the spread of the sickle gene would have been a relatively slow process, compared with the influence of traders, who transported large numbers of slaves over great distances. Four old men from Kano in northern Nigeria, who had at one time participated actively in slave trade, related to M. J. Herskovits the route they traveled with their caravans—a journey of some 1,800 miles into what is now Ghana. There is evidence to suggest that such travels were made far back in antiquity, so that slave trade as well as migrations could have significantly influenced the rise of the sickle gene.[11]

Another factor that we have neglected, but which may have contributed to the rise of the sickle gene, is polygamy. As noted by a Ghanian specialist in sickle cell anemia, F. I. D. Konotey-Ahulu,

> Population geneticists in developed countries . . . completely ignore the role of polygamy in sickle cell disease by looking merely at gene frequency rather than at the total number of diseased children produced. Gene frequency might remain the same if polygamy were similarly practiced by individuals with the [sickle] trait and by normal homozygous [AA] individuals. However, the disease problem . . . increases many fold if [individuals with sickle] trait take many wives. Indeed, the argument that the abnormal gene frequency goes up with polygamy cannot be entirely dismissed, because one of the reasons that Africans acquire more wives is the death of children born to the first wife. Such deaths occur more commonly in children of men with trait genes who often continue to acquire more wives until they find one whose children do not die from *chwe-chweechwe*.[12]

Chwechweechwe is the name for a set of symptoms in the Ga language of Ghana that Konotey-Ahulu claims is the indigenous identification of sickle cell disease. Konotey-Ahulu suggests that the onomatopoetic quality of the word *chwechweechwe* reflects the "relentless, repetitive, gnawing" of the pain associated with sickle cell anemia.

While on the decline in many regions, polygamy is nevertheless still practiced widely in parts of tropical Africa. For example, it is not hard to find Igbo men today with two wives, but they appear to be in the minority and polygamy is far below the excesses of some of the famous chiefs such as Onyeama, who claimed 53 wives at the time of his death in 1933. While polygamy may have given the sickle gene an extra boost, it could not be the primary factor. Polygamy alone does not explain the appearance of enough AS individuals to produce the SS children whose deaths could have provoked men to take more wives. Therefore, we conclude that the influence of malaria must be the most important factor, as deduced from the striking geographical coincidence of regions where the sickle gene is prevalent and where malaria is endemic. Added to this is the convincing laboratory demonstration that the malaria parasite does not multiply as well in AS cells, particularly at low levels of oxygenation, as it does in AA cells (see Chapter 6).[13]

The predominant factor in the spread of the sickle gene to the Western Hemisphere was, of course, slave trade, which ruptured African societies and whose consequences still weigh heavily on black Americans. In the United States currently about 10% of the black community are carriers of sickle trait. Therefore, on the average, 1% (10% × 10%) of all black couples are at risk of having a homozygous SS child. For these heterozygous couples, on the average 1 child out of 4 will be afflicted with sickle cell anemia, that is, about 1 out of every 400 black children born in the United States. This incidence, which is far higher than for other known genetic diseases, has led to routine testing of newborns for sickle cell anemia in several states. One consequence of the relatively high levels of the sickle gene in the United States was that sickle cell anemia was recognized as a disease earlier than would otherwise have been the case. In the long run, efforts to develop a treatment for American blacks, currently led by the Sickle Cell Branch of the National Institutes of Health, will also benefit Africans with sickle cell disease.

The dimensions of the slavery holocaust are difficult to grasp. According to estimates summarized in the *Cambridge Encyclopedia of Africa,* in the period between 1701 and 1810 over 7 million slaves were exported from Africa to the Americas. According to firsthand accounts from the later years of the eighteenth century, approximately 16,000 Igbo alone were sold into slavery each year. The practice of slavery tore at the fabric of Igbo society, as the threats of kidnapping rose dramatically and prisoners taken in warfare were also increasingly likely to be sold into slavery. By the first half of the nineteenth century transatlantic slave trade had declined, and by 1830 the ports of the Niger delta were ceasing to export slaves, as Great Britain and then other nations took active measures to eliminate slavery. Nevertheless, the corrupting effects of slave commerce remained with the Igbos for some time. One of the most unfortunate consequences was the disregard for human life bred by the slave trade, as evidenced by human sacrifices during burial ceremonies for important persons. While the practices probably predate transatlantic slave trade, the rituals reached incredible proportions, particularly in the period of "surplus" when the external markets for slaves were disappearing. According to E. Isichei, 40 slaves were killed at the burial of the leader Obi Ossah in 1845, with the surplus of slaves reaching such levels that by 1880 the rate of exchange was one horse for four to six adult slaves. Overall, slavery was a practice that decimated the population and diverted energy from more durable economic activities. According to some observers, the retarded economic development of equatorial Africa that has persisted into the twentieth century can be laid at the feet of the slave trade. The particular horrors associated with the transatlantic passage have also been thoroughly documented.[14]

Once the Igbo slaves reached the Americas, most traces of Igbo ethnic identity appear to have been lost in the caldron of slave commerce. This disappearance contrasts with other ethnic groups, such as the Yoruba, who have left a clearer legacy that includes relatively intact communities, notably in Cuba. Nevertheless, a 1794 history of the British colonies in the Americas by B. Edwards includes a description of slaves belonging to a group called the "Eboes." In addition to the stereotypical and deprecating remarks typical of the period, the author states that "if their confidence be once obtained, they manifest as great fidelity, affection and gratitude as can reasonably be expected from men in a state of slavery." In support of the identification of these "Eboes" as the Igbos of Nigeria is Edwards' observation that these people "universally practice circumcision"—a practice prevalent to this day among the Igbos. Melville J. Herskovits has also summarized some of the particular characteristics reported for Igbo slaves in the New World, including a relatively high degree of suicide which, he observed, reflected the "sensitive and independent spirit" of these people.[15]

Few additional clues are available to link any slaves to their Igbo roots. Early lists of American slaves assembled by Newbell Puckett include a small number of given names, some of which coincide with entries in the *Dictionary of Igbo Names* compiled by John Njoko. These include:

Name	Gender	Meaning
Aba	Female	Branch
Acha	Male	Best
Ada	Female	First daughter of family
Chima	Male	God knows
Lolo	Female	Woman priest
Onah	Male	Homeward

Slave lists in America indicate a marked decline in African names during the nineteenth century. According to Newbell Puckett, a quarter of the male slaves in the eighteenth century had names that were recognizably African, but "by the mid-nineteenth century less than one-half of one percent of all names collected suggest the possibility of African origin."[16]

Even in Igbo territory, the traditional names are being replaced in large measure by Christian names. Among the *ogbanje* children at the Awgu school, nearly half had names commonly found in any American elementary school: Caroline, Elizabeth, Felix, Vincent. The remainder had Igbo names. Some I am not able to translate, but the following occur in Njoko's dictionary:

Name	Gender	Meaning
Chibue	Male	God is king
Onuchukwu	Male	Spokesman of God
Ngosika	Female	Blessing is greater

The influence of Christian missionaries, reflected in the partial abandoning of traditional names, may have also served to mask traditional responses to sickle cell disease, but—as will be discussed in the following chapter—not entirely.

In summary, we may conclude that the sickle mutation occurred a few thousand years ago, and rose in incidence owing to natural selection assisted by other factors, including voluntary and involuntary migration. At the time that the sickle mutation began to spread, the transition from hunting and gathering to sedentary farming societies was occurring on a widening scale. The introduction of root crops such as yams led to the slash-and-burn cultivation that provides breeding sites for the *Anopheles* mosquito which transmits malaria. The spread of this disease ultimately led to the selection of sickle cell trait. The replacement of a single amino acid would have remained innocuous—existing almost exclusively in the heterozygous state in a small fraction of the population, as happens for most of the hundreds of other hemoglobin mutations discovered—were it not for malaria. By retarding growth of the malaria parasite, the sickle gene provided its possessors with a slight advantage over noncarriers, such that about 10% more survived to pass on their genes to the next generation. This advantage of AS individuals over AA individuals was almost certainly too small to be noticed by the Africans in whom this slow statistical game was being played.

While the analysis of the rise of AS individuals presented here is consistent with information from several sources, it does leave one perplexing question. Why did the sickle mutation appear in large numbers of individuals in Africa, but not in other parts of the world where malaria is endemic? The latest evidence (to be presented in Chapter 7) indicates that the sickle gene arose at least three times in Africa, whereas in the Mediterranean basin, different mutations involving the loss of the beta chain of hemoglobin arose and reached appreciable frequencies as a response, presumably, to malaria. When beta chain deficiencies occur in the homozygous state, a disease called beta-thalassemia is produced which often has more severe consequences than sickle cell anemia. Why sickle cell anemia should have predominated in Africa and beta-thalassemia in the Mediterranean basin is an intriguing mystery.

One possible explanation for the unique appearance of the sickle mutation in Africa concerns the role of diet. Linda Jackson has called attention to cassava, or manioc (*Manihot esculenta, Crantz*), which is one of the main staples for many African peoples and contains chemicals that can spontaneously liberate cyanate.

As discussed more fully in a later chapter, cyanate was one of the first compounds investigated as an antisickling agent for use in treating individuals with sickle cell anemia. Jackson's studies in Liberia have revealed that although malaria is encountered uniformly in different regions of the country, the incidence of the sickle gene is uneven, with lower values found in areas where cassava is regularly consumed. Although migrations could be responsible, an effect of diet may also be involved.

Cyanate from dietary sources could have influence on either sickling or malaria (and perhaps both). According to laboratory studies, cyanate inhibits growth of the malaria parasite, *Plasmodium falciparum*. Earlier work had established that cyanate inhibits sickling by reacting directly with hemoglobin. On the basis of these results, Jackson has proposed two ways that cassava consumption may have influenced the distribution of the sickle mutation. On the one hand, where cassava is consumed regularly in large quantities, the antimalarial effects of the cyanate may minimize the advantage of the sickle mutation. If the malaria incidence is partially reduced by diet, less of an advantage for survival with the hemoglobin S mutation would be expected for AS individuals as compared with AA individuals. This effect would explain the lower incidence of AS individuals among cassava consumers. On the other hand, sporadic consumption may lead to a modification of the hemoglobin S by cyanate that counteracts sickling, thereby increasing the fitness of the homozygous SS individuals. While this effect would not explain why lower levels of the sickle gene are found in regions with high cassava consumption, it might, according to Jackson, explain why the sickle mutation arose only in Africa, if a dietary factor is responsible.[17]

Unfortunately for this argument, cassava was introduced from South America by traders only a few hundred years ago, well after the sickle mutation was widespread, so it is probably not the dietary factor responsible for the spread of the sickle gene. The yam, on the other hand, a traditional foodstuff of many West Africans and a plant that has probably been cultivated for thousands of years in the region, is a better candidate. In an analysis of factors that might influence the incidence of the sickle mutation in many different ethnic groups, William Durham found a strong correlation between high S levels and yam consumption, once the data were adjusted for average rainfall. The rainfall favors growth of the *Anopheles* mosquito that transmits the malaria parasite, and therefore the selective advantage of the S mutation is greater in regions of heavy rainfall. In general, rainfall is limited to a short wet season, during which a burst of mosquitos appears, since they require ponds for reproduction. In some regions there are two closely spaced rainy periods, but a peak of mosquito growth occurs only in the first. While in general the incidence of the S gene is greater in regions of more abundant rainfall, for comparable levels of rainfall the incidence of the S gene is higher for yam-consuming peoples (generally ethnic groups with languages in the Kwa class of Niger-Congo languages), as compared with rice-consuming peoples.

One possible explanation for the higher frequency of the sickle mutation among yam eaters is the effect of cyanates or other chemicals from yam that interact with hemoglobin. If the severity of sickling among SS individuals were reduced in this way, the Fitness(SS) would be raised and the percentage of AS individuals would consequently increase. One difficulty with this argument is that the same effect could diminish the properties of AS cells that help them resist malaria. Thus, even though the numbers of AS individuals born would increase, their reproductive fitness would decrease. Nevertheless, African populations could have the best of both effects, if they abstained from eating yams during the peak weeks of mosquito infestation. The ability of AS cells to resist malaria would not be diminished during the most critical period, and for the rest of the year yam consumption could improve the condition of SS individuals. Perhaps African societies have achieved this ideal, since as Durham states, "I find it provocative, therefore, to note that the consumption of new yams [the first of each year's crop] is sternly prohibited among virtually all the Kwa yam growers until after the first of the annual rainfall peaks, and the only malaria peak, has passed." Indeed, one of the major social events of the year for many African societies is the yam festival celebrating the moment when the new yams may be consumed.[18]

While the role of yams in the diet could help explain the incidence of the S gene in a population, it does not directly explain why the S mutation was selected in Africa because of its antimalarial effects, whereas beta-thalassemia arose in the malarious

Mediterranean basin. Moreover, the latest results with cyanate indicate that it is a very weak antisickling agent in vivo. Therefore, if a specific factor is present in yams, chemicals of an entirely different class may be involved.

An additional set of clues as to the nature of these chemicals comes from another deficiency of red blood cells, but one that does not involve hemoglobin. Certain populations around the world show a deficiency of the enzyme glucose-6-phosphate dehydrogenase, but their distribution is less clearly related to malaria than is the sickle mutation. In 1976 Huheey and Martin proposed that a deficiency of this enzyme does provide resistance to malaria, but only when fava beans are part of the diet. Ingestion of fava beans (*Vicia fava*) can cause red cell hemolysis, a condition known as favism which is particularly common in Mediterranean and Middle East countries. Apparently fava contains strong oxidizing agents that are normally neutralized in a series of reactions involving the enzyme glucose-6-phosphate dehydrogenase. Moreover, the *Plasmodium* parasites responsible for malaria are particularly sensitive to oxidizing agents. Even normal oxygen levels inhibit their growth, and a key to successful laboratory cultivation of the parasites in red cells is to diminish oxygen levels. Therefore, for individuals deficient in glucose-6-phosphate dehydrogenase, the active agents in fava, while causing favism in extreme cases, may provide a natural protection against malaria by releasing oxidizing agents. This theory has received strong confirmation recently by Golenser and co-workers, who have demonstrated a direct inhibition of *Plasmodium falciparum* development by the agent from fava, isouramil, but only when the parasites are grown in cells deficient in glucose-6-phosphate.[19]

The connections among favism, glucose-6-phosphate, and malaria suggest that any changes which create a more oxidizing environment in the red cell may impede development of the malaria parasite. Indeed, an explanation along these lines is suspected for beta-thalassemia, involving oxidation of iron in the excess hemoglobin alpha chains, accompanied by production of highly reactive oxygen radicals and superoxides. In the case of sickle cell hemoglobin, a direct effect of this type is less obvious, but various disruptions of cellular equilibria caused by membrane deformations and damage associated with sickling could have similar effects. In this case as well, dietary factors may play a decisive role in determining which type of mutation is likely to be selected for its antimalarial effects. The extensive analysis by B. Ames of strong oxidizing compounds found in food illustrates that there is no shortage of candidates for possible agents that could influence red cell oxidation, in conjunction with red cell enzyme or hemoglobin deficiencies.[20]

Overall, we cannot say with certainty whether or not diet played a specific role in the evolution of sickling cells. A great deal more information will be necessary to settle this matter. What we do know is that, with or without a dietary mechanism, eventually the AS individuals in tropical Africa reached large enough percentages of their respective populations that marriages between two AS individuals became increasingly common and resulted in the birth of some SS children. The sickle gene can be thought of as a natural form of chemotherapy against malaria which, although modestly successful, has a latent side effect that appears only in subsequent generations. In this case, the side effect is the appearance of disease in homozygous SS children. That they were born in large numbers, we can be sure. Since 25% of the Igbo are carriers, 6% (25% × 25%) of all couples consist of parents who are both carriers, and one in four of their children, or 1.5% of all Igbo children born, will be homozygous SS. At the same time, we know that children throughout history died in large numbers from many causes, with the pattern of high infant mortality being reversed only in this century and only in more medically advanced societies. Therefore, the question is now squarely framed: Were Africans generally aware of sickle cell anemia before its discovery in the United States, and if so, how did they respond?

CHAPTER 4

AFRICAN REPEATER
CHILDREN

From our glimpse into the past, we have reconstructed several stages in the history of human evolution and sickle cell anemia. A remaining issue to be considered is the extent to which Africans perceived and specifically identified the consequences of sickling cells in their bloodstreams. Were the *ogbanje* children in the Awgu school the end result of a chain of events that was initiated with a single mutation in the DNA, one that caused red cells to sickle and to impinge on a segment of the human population which, in turn, explained these experiences largely on the basis of animistic concepts? These possible linkages were continually on my mind as I crossed the soft rolling hills between the lodgings in Enugu and the Awgu school. There were scores of walkers along the road, mainly women with enormous loads carried on their heads—a bundle of firewood, a large water jug, or sometimes a tub of produce on the way to market—women who had perhaps suffered the repeated deaths of their children from sickle cell disease.

One of the first goals of this study was to obtain blood samples from the *ogbanje* children and their parents in order to test for hemoglobin S. The efforts to arrange for blood samples required several visits; with each one, more information and deeper insights into the *ogbanje* tradition were obtained. We discovered that these children, with one exception, were not born missing a portion of their finger (as was "one of the stubborn ones" described by

Achebe and quoted in Chapter 1). The ends of the left little fingers of these children had been amputated in the first year or two of their lives as part of a ritual to induce them to "stay," once they had been identified as *ogbanjes*. A scar was clearly visible at the site of the amputation for all but one of the children. The one exception, Onuchukwu, was born, according to his parents, with an incomplete little finger. In addition, he was born missing both small toes. We learned that toes rather than fingers are sometimes cut in *ogbanje* rituals. In fact, the left fourth toe of the mother of one of the Awgu *ogbanje* children had been removed because she herself was suspected of being an *ogbanje*. We shall see that birth defects of the type that Onuchukwu experienced may have played an important role in the origins of the *ogbanje* practices.

The traditional Igbo belief is that children are normally the reincarnation of deceased ancestors, although in the Igbo view an independent existence is maintained by the spirit of the deceased ancestor apart from the child. Therefore, it is possible to find several children of a clan who are identified as the reincarnation of the same ancestor. In this respect, the African concept of reincarnation differs from familiar Asian concepts, which show a one-to-one correspondence between a deceased individual and a newborn.

Igbo people place particular importance on the association of a child with a deceased person, claiming that the child will be restless until the identification is made. Therefore, traditional Igbo parents consult a diviner after the birth of each child to identify the reincarnating ancestor. Then, at least in the Awka region studied by Glen Webb, a carved wooden effigy, called an *okpenshi*, represents the reincarnating ancestor and is consecrated by the sacrifice of a chicken. "For the rest of the child's life, this *okpenshi* will serve as the medium through which the reincarnating ancestor is intermittently given oblations on the child's behalf (and later by the grown child himself, in the case of a male) in the effort to insure the spirit's cooperation in fostering his current manifestation's well-being." Among African styles of statuary art, the *okpenshi* is a remarkably abstract representation of an ancestor (see Fig. 4.1).

When an Igbo woman marries, she moves to the compound of her husband's family and may have only infrequent contact with her original family. Therefore, when a child is born, a deceased

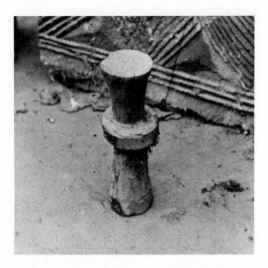

Figure 4.1. *Okpenshi* statue. (From N. Neaher.)

relative from the father's side is more likely to be a candidate for the reincarnating ancestor.[1] According to Igbo beliefs, the return of an ancestor is sometimes prevented when a malevolent spirit displaces an ancestor in a newborn. These spirits, it is said, are malevolent because they are born with the intention of dying early. They come to human existence briefly to torment the parents, while retaining ties to the spirit world that will pull them back long before they have led a full life. According to Dr. M. Ogbolu Okonji, one of the few modern social scientists to write about *ogbanje:*

> The word *ogbanje* in ordinary Igbo usage means one who makes frequent and regular trips. The religious notion being discussed here has this same meaning, but in addition also refers to a condition of existence and the symbol of that condition. Thus it refers to an individual who goes through a continuous circle of birth and death as a result of a sort of primeval oath (*iyi uwa:* oath of the world) taken in the spirit world in the presence of the creator and binding on the living. The oath is believed to be binding on the one who has taken it: the individual has to live in a particular manner throughout his or her usually short span of life. The object for the oath is hidden away from ordinary human sight and usually buried under a huge tree, in the person's palm, or in other impressive places. It seems that all those who have sworn this kind of oath and are therefore

ogbanje, are linked in some sort of spiritual kinship: they tend to, or rather are believed to behave in a similar manner and are believed always to be in sympathy or communicate telepathically with one another—all these without being conscious of any sort of special relationship with one another except when under the spell of some charms.

According to Igbo traditions, *ogbanje* children return repeatedly to the same parents. They die prematurely, only to arrive again with the birth of the next child. As in Achebe's narrative, Igbo people speak of cases where the cycle is repeated again and again, six, seven, eight, or even nine times. Parents begin to suspect that they are plagued by a "repeater child" if they have suffered the deaths of several children and especially if each death precedes the birth of the next child. This next child is then thought to be a living *ogbanje* and dramatic action to protect its death is considered. An "*ogbanje* doctor" may be consulted and serious measures may be proposed, as in the ceremony described by Okonji:

> The arrangements are often elaborate and expensive. The rites are often excruciating, in fact a nightmare for the patient. The form of the ritual does vary from practitioner to practitioner. But the medicine pot that is placed upon the head of the patient and the music are the constant features of the ceremony. The frenzied drum beat, the dizzy dance of the *ogbanje* who swerves back and forth with the medicine pot on the head unsupported with the hand and yet steady, all tend to lend credence to the claim that the *ogbanje* doctor's skill or art has some supernatural origin. The drumming and the dancing set the mood of the ceremony. But what seem to be most important are the chalk powder and the thick stew of herbal concoction that are showered on the *ogbanje,* for without their at once soothing and stimulating influences, the patient cannot acquire the extrasensory perceptual powers by means of which the object on which the oath was sworn can be perceived. It is the initiate who points out the spot where the object has been buried . . . When the spot where the object for the oath is buried has been located, the whole surrounding [area] is excavated. By careful searching, by means of the doctor's spells and dexterity, the object may be found. Usually it is a well-polished pebble or a beautifully-threaded bunch of cowries or coral beads or other impressive objects. Whether what is found has been put there by the doctor himself or not is another question. What is important is that the ritual does

seem to perform some function for the personality adjustment of the individual and the family concerned.[2]

Other measures include the drastic step of cutting the little finger. What this amputation is to accomplish lies hidden within mythic tradition. One *ogbanje* doctor explained that the *ogbanje* spirits are a vain cult and any disfigurement causes rejection by the group. In this way, *ogbanje* children will not be called back to join their peers in the spirit world after a brief sojourn in the world of the living. They will be ignored and permitted to remain with their parents.

The day for our obtaining blood samples finally arrived. To help reassure the villagers, who were unaccustomed to giving blood, the help of Richard Tagbo, an Igbo technician from the University of Nigeria Teaching Hospital in Enugu, had fortunately been secured. His skill in obtaining samples quickly, even from young children, and his ability to persuade villagers to participate in our research guaranteed the success of our efforts. We set up shop in a corner of the school and obtained blood samples from 8 of the original *ogbanje* school children, as well as 5 pre-school children living in the vicinity of the school who also had had the ends of their little fingers removed (Fig. 4.2). In addition, blood samples were obtained from 8 of the parents of the *ogbanje*

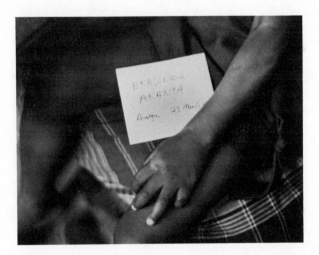

Figure 4.2. An *ogbanje* child with an amputated left little finger.

children. The children's family histories revealed that their births typically had been preceded by two or three siblings that died soon after birth.

In the laboratory, each individual's hemoglobins were migrated in an electric field to distinguish the forms A and S (or any other abnormalities). Results indicated that the *ogbanjes'* hemoglobin was, on the average, no different from the hemoglobin of other Igbos. Of the 13 *ogbanje* children whose left little fingers were, in the terminology of anatomists, missing the distal phalanx, 10 possessed only hemoglobin A, while the remaining 3 possessed both hemoglobin A and hemoglobin S. Therefore, the children were typical of the general Igbo population, which Lehmann and Nwokolo characterized in 1959 as having a 25% incidence of sickle trait (AS), on the basis of finding 64 traits in a sample of 257. Moreover, the parents we tested were also typical of the general Igbo population. Of the 8 parents tested, 6 were AA and 2 were AS.

According to a hypothesis which would directly link sickle cell anemia with the *ogbanje,* the deceased siblings of the living *ogbanje* children should have been mainly homozygous SS individuals who had died as a result of sickle cell anemia. For this to have been the case, however, both parents of the deceased child would have to possess the sickle gene. The *ogbanje* children we tested could be AA or AS (although a percentage of AS closer to 50% would have been expected, if both parents were AS), but in order for their deceased siblings to have died from sickle cell anemia, each parent should have been AS (or, though less likely, SS). Therefore, the finding that 6 out of 8 parents of the *ogbanje* children were AA eliminated in most cases sickle cell disease as the cause of the deceased siblings' deaths.

I had suspected, however, that the *ogbanje* children from the Awgu school could not be linked directly to sickle cell disease, even before the hemoglobin samples had been analyzed. There were simply too many *ogbanjes*. The 10 *ogbanje* children we first observed were in a school of about 200 children. Since the incidence of AS individuals in the Igbo population is 25%, the number of Igbo couples at risk for having a child with sickle cell disease is 1 in 16 couples (25% $\times$ 25%). Since on the average only 1 in 4 of the children for the couples at risk would be homozygous

SS individuals, in the population at large only 1 child in 64 would be expected to have sickle cell anemia. Thus, the level of sickle cell anemia in the general population is too low (about 1.5% of all newborns, with a significant number dying in the preschool age range) to be reconciled with a finding of about 5% *ogbanje* children in the Awgu school.

For these reasons, it is clear that among Igbo villagers in Awgu, a precise connection between sickle cell anemia and *ogbanje* does not always exist. However, it would be unrealistic to expect the Igbo to deliver foolproof diagnoses on the basis of the indirect symptoms that accompany sickle cell anemia, particularly in a region of extremely high infant mortality from many sources. A more likely explanation of the finger-shortening ritual is that sickle cell anemia could have historically given rise to the *ogbanje* concept; but once the concept was widespread in the traditions of the culture, its application became imprecise.

Igbo physicians trained in modern medicine were among the first to recognize the connection between *ogbanje* and sickle cell anemia, but without considering the two to be always tightly connected. For example, C. Nwokolo in a 1960 article commented: "I should like to express my belief that the widespread Ibo belief in 'ogbanje', that is the concept of children who come to the world again and again only to die, breaking their parents' hearts with a sadistic regularity, probably arises from the widespread existence of sickle cell anemia, and suggests that the disease must have been with our ancestors for many generations."[3] This article is probably the earliest suggestion of a link between *ogbanje* and sickle cell anemia. The theme was taken up again in 1983 by J. Onwubalili. In response, data on the Awgu children were presented to demonstrate that the connection is not always clear cut. Onwubalili replied that because practices may also vary in different parts of Nigeria, the possibility that a more solid connection between sickle cell and *ogbanje* exists elsewhere should be explored.[4]

If such a connection even among other groups cannot be established at the present time, it nevertheless appears highly plausible that *ogbanje* practices were originally linked to sickle cell anemia, at least in part. One of the common early symptoms of sickle cell anemia is painful swelling in the joints, particularly those of the

hand, which may lead to bone infections. When a finger or toe is
visibly affected, the condition is called dactylitis. As noted by
Bunn and his coauthors,

> Dactylitis may be the initial symptom of SS disease in infants. It is
> characterized by the rather sudden onset over hours to a day or two
> of painful swelling of the dorsum of both hands and feet. Usually at
> least two and frequently all four extremities are involved. Dactylitis
> may occur before the first year of age and generally does not occur
> after the age of 5. Children with dactylitis usually have fever and, as
> might be expected, irritability. A single episode may last for one to
> two weeks and may recur one or more times during the next several
> months or years.[5]

According to Serjeant and Ashcroft, the dactylitis associated
with sickle cell anemia can interfere with the development of the
hand and result in one exceptionally short finger (Fig. 4.3). At
some time in the past the Igbos may have recognized a condition
(what we now know to be sickle cell disease) in which a number of

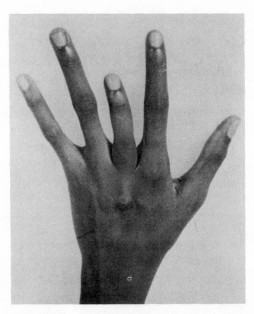

Figure 4.3. A miniature finger on the hand of an adult with sickle cell anemia.
(From O. Akinyanju.)

children in a particular family died. If the surviving child was one of the occasional homozygous SS individuals with a miniature finger, the conclusion may have been drawn that a short finger was necessary for survival. As a consequence of this belief, families experiencing the consecutive deaths of children may have applied the finger-shortening ritual. At the same time, the idea that *ogbanje* spirits dislike disfigured bodies may also have become associated with this ritual. It is noteworthy that just as dactylitis strikes both fingers and toes, *ogbanje* rituals involve the amputation or partial amputation of toes as well as fingers.

Another possible explanation of the finger-cutting ritual concerns the fact that pain and swelling in the hands and fingers are often the first symptoms of sickle cell anemia. Cutting a finger may have corresponded to some elementary notion of purging a noxious agent at the site of the irritation. Further evidence that the first *ogbanjes* may have been victims of sickle cell anemia comes from the fact that both *ogbanjes* and victims of the disease are considered (in the eyes of the Igbos) to be especially beautiful. As pointed out in Chapter 1, this beauty may have been attributable to the distorted skull that characterizes many victims of sickle cell anemia.

But before such links can be asserted, the question must be addressed whether the Igbos and other peoples of tropical Africa ever possessed an awareness of sickle cell anemia as a discrete disease. Certainly if they did not, there could be no connection between the disease and the *ogbanje* rituals. According to the Ghanaian specialist on sickle cell disease, Konotey-Ahulu, many African ethnic groups *were* aware of the specific symptoms of sickle cell anemia and had special names describing them. Konotey-Ahulu has compiled a list of indigenous terms for sickle cell anemia from many parts of West Africa.

Name	*Language*
Chwechweechwe	Ga
Hemkom	Adangme, Krobo, Shai, Ada
Ahotutuo	Twi, Akan, Akwapim
Nuidudui or Chichi	Ewe
Nwiiwii or Kwaha	Fante
Dobakotiri	Dagbani
Amosani	Hausa

Name	Language
Koba-Tuem	Buili
Paa	Kassena-Nankani
Itaangmi	Bassari (Togo)
Dongadonga	Northern Togo dialect
Lakuregbee	Yoruba
Orengua	Isokko
Aju-oyi	Ibo, Item
Adep	Banyangi (Cameroon)

A family of the Krobo group in Ghana can trace sickle cell disease back to 1670 in 9 successive generations, according to Konotey-Ahulu. While such exceptionally accurate diagnoses may have occurred occasionally, I doubt that they were common. Sickle cell disease was superimposed, after all, onto a background of many childhood illnesses and high infant mortality from a number of infectious diseases, including malaria. The names cited above may have been applied to illnesses from a variety of sources. For example, the Igbo word cited by Konotey-Ahulu, *aju-oyi*, means serious illness, according to native speakers, and is not generally regarded by the Igbo to be specific for sickle cell disease. Therefore, for various ethnic groups, an answer to the question whether they reliably recognized sickle cell disease must remain incomplete.[6]

Once the results from my initial attempt to find an indigenous African response to sickle cell anemia were obtained, I realized that much more work was necessary to reach a firm conclusion. Since sickle cell anemia is prevalent across the African tropics, information was needed on how widespread the belief in *ogbanje*-like phenomena might be. It was clear that the investigations should be broadened to include other African ethnic groups and to explore the possible impact of sickle cell disease on their cultures. In addition, the occurrence of birthmarks of the type possessed by Onuchukwu raised the issue of the possible role birthmarks played in the origin of the *ogbanje* concept and also in the more general African belief in reincarnation.

The idea of "repeater children" is not unique to the Igbo. A number of other ethnic groups in Africa have similar beliefs. Among the Yoruba, a large ethnic group of southwestern Nigeria, children known as *àbíkú* share many similarities with the *ogbanje* children of the Igbo. In his book on the Yoruba, Bascom notes that the Yoruba believe all children are manifestations of reincarnated ancestors. This belief is so prevalent that male children are commonly named Babatunde (which means "father returns") and female children are commonly named Yetunde (which means "mother returns"). Prior to being reborn, each soul, according to Yoruba tradition, appears before Olorun, the Sky God, to arrange its new destiny.

If a woman has several children in succession who die at childbirth, in infancy, or even when somewhat older, they may not be several different ancestral souls, but one ancestral soul being repeatedly reborn only to return shortly to heaven where it retains its childlike form. It has been granted short spans of life by Olorun because it does not want to remain long on earth, preferring life in heaven or wishing only to travel back and forth between heaven and earth. Such children are known as *àbikú* or "one born to die"; in a society where infant mortality is high, *àbikú* are common.

Parents may have charms made to keep an *àbikú* from leaving them or they may be told by a *babalawo* [diviner-priest] to make a sacrifice or to have the child worship a particular deity. In Meko and Igana the mother may join a cult group which propitiates *àbikú* and has large iron rattles made for the child to wear on its ankles. Sometimes the corpse of a child is marked by shaving a spot on its head or cutting a notch in its ear so as to prove it is an *àbikú* when it is reborn with the same mark. Sometimes a corpse of an *àbikú* is threatened with burning or with the cutting off of a toe or finger to frighten it into staying on earth when it is reborn again.[7]

Just as novels dealing with Igbo life have helped elaborate the *ogbanje* concept, so too the *àbikú* child has been described in detail. For instance, the eloquent Yoruba writer Wole Soyinka, recollecting his childhood, writes,

The bookseller's wife was one of our many mothers ... Her only daughter, Bukola, was not of our world. When we threw our voices against the school walls of Lower Parsonage and listened to them echo from a long distance, it seemed to me that Bukola was one of the denizens of that other world where the voice was caught, sieved, re-spun and cast back in diminished copies. Amulets, bangles, tiny rattles and dark copper-twist rings earthed her through ankles, fingers, wrists and waist. She knew she was *àbikú* (a child which is born, dies, is born again and dies in a repetitive cycle). The two tiny cicatrices on her face were also part of the many counters to enticements by her companions in the other world. Like all *àbikú* she was privileged, apart. Her parents dared not scold her for long or earnestly.[8]

The Yoruba concept of *àbikú* closely resembles the Igbo concept of *ogbanje*. Moreover, the Yoruba have a level of sickle cell trait in the population comparable to that of the Igbo; thus, the *àbikú* concept, like the *ogbanje* concept, could have some relationship to sickle cell anemia. Efforts were made during trips to Nigeria to find *àbikú* children and their parents who might be tested for sickle cell hemoglobin. We obtained secondhand reports of *àbikú* and met a number of adults who claimed to have been *àbikú*, with birthmarks alleged to correspond to burns inflicted on the cadaver of a preceding deceased sibling. However, efforts to establish close relationships with village groups in order to study their children were not fruitful. On several occasions, Yoruba contacts who were accustomed to interacting with Americans or Europeans offered to provide introductions in villages or families where *àbikú* children were found. But in each case, as the time for making contact neared, the offer was withdrawn and always for the same reason. The contact person feared that any difficulty befalling the villagers after our visit—an illness, accident, or other misfortune—would be blamed on the visit of Caucasians, and the Yoruba person who arranged the meeting ultimately would be held responsible. This possibility posed too great a risk. Overall, the Yoruba were less willing than the Igbo to discuss such matters with outsiders.

The reluctance of Yoruba villagers to discuss their traditions with outsiders is symptomatic of the prevailing African idea that events are being shaped by apparently indirect causes. The openness that we encountered among the Igbo proves to be the exception, perhaps because, as stressed by Ottenberg, the Igbo "are probably most receptive to culture change, and most willing to accept Western ways, of any large group in Nigeria." Ottenberg cites a number of historical and cultural reasons for this fact.[9] However, the important conclusion to be drawn from the Yoruba is that their concerns about undesirable consequences from unusual events reveal much about African notions of magic and witchcraft and the common sources of misfortune. In discussing the Azande of Central Africa, Evans-Prichard captures the sense of subtle causes inherent in the natural philosophy of witchcraft.

As a natural philosophy it reveals a theory of causation. Misfortune is due to witchcraft cooperating with natural forces. If a buffalo gores a man, or the supports of a granary are undermined by termites so that it falls on his head, or he is infected with cerebrospinal meningitis, Azande say that the buffalo, the granary, and the disease, are causes which combine with witchcraft to kill a man. Witchcraft does not create the buffalo and the granary and the disease for these exist in their own right, but it is responsible for the particular situation in which they are brought into lethal relations with a particular man. The granary would have fallen in any case, but since there was witchcraft present it fell at the particular moment when a certain man was resting beneath it. Of these causes the only one which permits intervention is witchcraft, for witchcraft emanates from a person. The buffalo and the granary do not allow of intervention and are, therefore, whilst recognized as causes, not considered the socially relevant ones.[10]

It is possible that investigators who could spend longer periods with the Yoruba would eventually overcome the villagers' fears of witchcraft and successfully complete studies of the *àbikú*. Despite our own inability to do so, information obtained from various sources verifies the existence of a strongly held Yoruba belief in *àbikú* that parallels the Igbo belief in *ogbanje*. In fact, the Yoruba concept may even be the more highly developed of the two, as evidenced by a particular form of statuette related to *àbikú* rituals (Fig. 4.4; the vessel was believed to be used as a receptacle for gifts to induce the *àbikú* to "stay") and by a lengthy list of Yoruba names specifically assigned to *àbikú* children.[11]

A brief period of field work in Benin City revealed that the Edo—another Nigerian ethnic group with many features in common with the Yoruba—also believe in repeater children, whom they call *igbankhuan*. One adult woman was introduced to us as an *igbankhuan* who was induced to stay. The woman had an *igbankhuan* name, Awurhio, meaning one who dies and rises. Awurhio, like the *àbikú* individuals described earlier, had a birthmark on her abdomen said to correspond to burns inflicted on the cadaver of her preceding sibling.

According to published reports, the Efiks of southern Nigeria also identify "repeater babies," known in their language as *ekabasi*. Similarly, Talbot noted that among the Ibibio, neighbors of the Igbo, "if one child after another dies in a family—or as most peoples here say 'the child keeps on dying,' since it is thought to

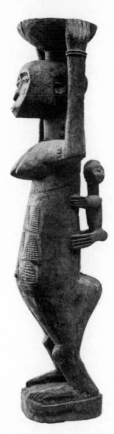

Figure 4.4. *Àbíkú* statuette described by Merlo, 1975. (From Musée de l'Homme.)

be the same soul trying to incarnate—a finger or toe is cut off or the body burnt, so that the troublesome visitor may leave the mother in peace."[12] Verger cites *danwabi* as the term that the Hausa (the major northern Nigerian ethnic group) apply to repeater children.

It gradually became apparent to me that a belief in repeater children characterizes many of the ethnic groups of southern Nigeria, and I began to explore how far beyond Nigeria the belief could be found. Many African myths extend with remarkable similarity over great geographical distances. For example, a common African myth concerning the origin of death, designated by J. G. Frazer as "the tale of two messengers," appears this way in the Igbo version:

God sent the dog who was his head messenger to men with the message that if anyone died, the body should lie upon the earth and be strewn with ashes, after which the dead person would come back to life. The dog was delayed by hunger and tiredness, so God sent a sheep with the same message. The sheep, too, stopped on the way in order to eat, and when it arrived it had forgotten the wording of the message, and said to men that a person who had died was to be buried in the earth. When, now, the dog arrived with the right message, he was not believed and he was told "we have already received the word from the creator by the sheep that all dead bodies should be buried."[13]

Variations on the tale of two messengers among diverse African ethnic groups involve different animals. The most common version, found in Nigeria among the Hausa, involves a chameleon as the first messenger and a lizard as the second. This chameleon–lizard version extends as far as the Zulu of East Africa. For the Ashanti of Ghana, the myth is based on a goat followed by a sheep, while for the Bongo the same animals are used as in the Igbo version but their roles are reversed. Other animals that appear in the same basic motif include a cat, spider, tortoise, hen, frog, duck, hyena, mole, and centipede.

It is clear from the tale of two messengers, also known as "the message that failed," that mythic ideas often have a wide diffusion in Africa. Such myths could have been transmitted across linguistic barriers by bilingual individuals, especially in regions where different ethnic groups inhabit adjacent territories and where bilingualism is common. In addition, Africans often possess knowledge of the principal language of commerce of each major region of Africa, as well as their mother tongue. Alternatively, the myths may be so old that they were transmitted from one generation to the next before languages evolved to become mutually unintelligible. Either explanation also could apply to the belief in repeater children. As I accumulated more information, it became apparent that the belief in repeater children exists among ethnic groups that are as widely separated geographically as the groups who believe in the tale of two messengers.

In attempting to define the geographical limits of the notion of repeater children, I found it relatively easy to establish the western boundary. It is the Atlantic Ocean. During field work carried out in Senegal, I encountered practices involving repeater children among the Wolof and Serer similar to those observed in Nigeria. Along the beautiful beaches of the western tip of Africa, I learned that the Wolof, who reside in the area surrounding Dakar, and the Serer, who live along the coast south of Dakar, both perform minor amputations, principally small cuts in the ear, on their presumed repeater children. While this ritual is generally applied to living children, the claim is also made that it is performed on cadavers of children and that subsequent children in the same family are born with corresponding cuts in their ears. In a village on the Senegal coast near Gambia, I met three adults with small pieces of the rims of their ears missing and heard stories of these incidents from older relatives, who claimed to have witnessed the marking of an earlier cadaver in the same way (Fig. 4.5).

H. Collomb translates the Serer term for repeater children, *tji:d a paxer,* as "the child who leaves and returns or the death of the same child." For the Serer,

> God, supreme force, generator of all life has created for man two bodies: one for the world of the living and one for the world of the dead. The one that is in the world of the dead functions as the matrix. All of the stigmas that mark the body in the world of the living (*anda*) also mark in the same way its double in the world of the dead (*alarira*). Children who depart quickly are marked in order to be recognized upon return. A part of the ear or finger is cut, a cut is

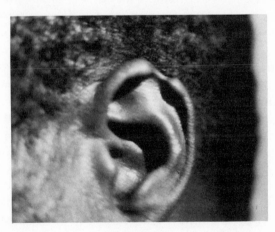

Figure 4.5. The ear of a young adult Serer male showing a notching typically associated with repeater children in Senegal.

made on the cheek or chest or a thorn is planted in the child's foot. Although, for all, the body of the child will decay in the earth, the double within *alarira* will bear the same mutilation and the new body it will engender will bear them also.[14]

Among the Serer, the sickle cell gene is found in a much smaller percentage of the population than in the Igbo or Yoruba: only 5% of the Serer are carriers of hemoglobin S.[15] For Collomb, the *tji:d a paxer* is more likely to be related to *kwashiorkor,* the syndrome of severe protein deficiency, than to sickle cell anemia.

From firsthand experience, it became evident to me that the concept of repeater children is a major element in the belief system of ethnic groups across the tropics of West Africa from Nigeria to Senegal. Also, while carrying out preliminary investigations among the Baoule of the Ivory Coast, I learned that repeater children are a part of that culture. In this case, a marking of the face occurred, on a cadaver according to my informants, or possibly on a living child, as suggested in Solinka's description of the cicatrices of the *àbíkú* child. In addition to my direct contacts, I began to delve into books and articles written about Africa in English and French, particularly by early visitors, to learn whether practices associated with repeater children were noted. I discovered that descriptions of the peoples of West Africa recount cadaver marking in many ethnic groups.[16]

While each ethnic group in West Africa has shaded the basic idea of repeater children to blend with its own traditions, the essential element of deceased children returning to the original mother is always present. In addition, the physical marking or mutilation of a child's body is widespread—either that of a living child or a cadaver. As for the presence of such beliefs in the tropics east of Nigeria, evidence was more difficult to obtain. Residents of Cameroon that I have met elsewhere in Africa have informed me that *ogbanje*-like practices are common among certain ethnic groups of their country; however, I have not had the opportunity to examine this myself and have not found any published reports. Among the published reports about East Africa that I have encountered, the passing on of particular physical characteristics from a deceased person to a child by reincarnation is believed by various East African peoples to occur. However, the phenomenon seems to be limited to characteristics passively acquired, in contrast to the deliberate marking of individuals or their cadavers as in West Africa. For example, a very early report from what is now Zaire discussing the belief in reincarnation notes: "Often particular children have a striking resemblance to a preceding incarnation and when an infant comes to the world with certain deformities, he is recognized as being the reincarnation of some recently deceased person who had been afflicted in the same way." Another early report from the region of Kenya follows a similar theme: "There is no particular taboo on crippled children, but the people say that the infant is the reincarnation of a deceased person similarly afflicted whom they remember, and give it his or her name."[17] From this and other reports, it appears that among the Bantu peoples beliefs similar to repeater children occur, but they have not become as intricate as those of West Africans, who believe that they can use markings to influence or monitor reincarnation.

While the occurrence of a belief in repeater children is a dominant feature on the cultural landscape of the western African tropics, more research among various ethnic groups is needed to determine whether repeater children have any connection with sickle cell anemia. In general, the occurrence of sickle cell anemia and the belief in repeater children overlap considerably in various ethnic groups, as indicated by Livingston's data on ethnic groups (in west to east order) identified as possessing a belief in repeater children. (For some population groups not identified ethnically, the designation by country is presented.)[18]

Ethnic Group	Sickle Trait
Serer	5%
Wolof	8%
Diola	13%
Bambara	11%
Baule	7%
Southern Ghana	17%
Yoruba	27%
Edo	29%
Cameroon (Yaounde)	20%
Congo (Kinshasa)	26%
baLuba	30%
Uganda	23%
Tanzania (Dar es Salaam)	13%
Kenya (incl. Kikuyu)	7%

The anatomical birth defects associated in some cases with repeater children also warrant additional investigation. In general, the birth defects alleged to correspond to the deliberate marking of a deceased relative would, of course, be expected to have more conventional causes, such as genetic abnormalities or traumas during pregnancy. But certain birth defects, such as the absence of a single bone of a finger, have no such known cause. There is a slight resemblance to cases of ectrodactyly (*ectro-* is a prefix from Greek roots meaning the congenital absence of a specified part) that have been described, but the loss of only the last digit of the left little finger, as observed for Onuchukwu, would be a most exceptional case of ectrodactyly.

In Nigeria, children born missing certain toes were also found, including Onuchukwu. Loss of toes is known to occur when the blood supply to a toe is cut off; atrophy and eventually autoamputation follow. However, S. G. Browne, who has studied this peculiarly tropical condition called ainhum, throughout the African equatorial region, notes that no cases have been observed in children under the age of 6 years; he also reports one patient with an ainhum-like condition of a finger. The fact that ainhum has not been found in young children, however, makes it unlikely to have played a role in children identified as repeaters.[19]

Whatever may prove to be the origin of the birthmarks and birth defects of repeater children, the beliefs surrounding these children are in my mind of great importance in understanding the origin of ancestor worship in Africa. This contrasts with the most common explanation of such traditions, derived from Tylor's line of argument, that dreams are responsible for the mythic view of the world that assigns control of events to spirits.

To understand the popular conceptions of the human soul or spirit, it is instructive to notice the words which have been found suitable to express it. The ghost or phantasm seen by the dreamer or the visionary is in unsubstantial form, like a shadow or reflection, and thus the familiar term of the *shade* comes in to express the soul. Thus the Tasmanian word for the shadow is also that of the spirit, the Algonquins describe a man's soul as *otachchuk*, 'his shadow'; the Quich language uses *natub* for 'shadow, soul'; the Arawak *ueja* means 'shadow, soul, image'; and Abipones made the one word *loakal* serve for 'shadow, soul, echo, image.' The Zulus not only use the word *tunzi* for 'shadow, spirit, ghost', but they consider that at death the

shadow of a man will in some way depart from the corpse, to become an ancestral spirit. The Basutos not only call the spirit remaining after death the *serit* or 'shadow', but they think that if a
man walks on the river bank, a crocodile may seize his shadow in
the water and draw him in; while in Old Calabar there is found the
same identification of the spirit with the *ukpon* or 'shadow', for a
man to lose which is fatal.[20]

Similar ideas were advanced by Delafosse. Others, such as Malinowski, give dreams less importance and view the doctrines about
souls and spirits as a form of wishful thinking which provides
emotional reassurance against the loss and dread of death. Yet
dreams currently occupy a primary role for traditional Africans,
with significance in a number of culturally important ways. For
example, Denise Paulme relates dreams and reincarnation for the
Kissi of Guinea. She describes the belief that each individual has
a shadow or double with soul-like attributes that is the active aspect of dreams.

> The term *wundule* designates something more than the projected
> shadow. The possession of the shadow, as that of the heart, is an es-
> sential condition of life. At death, the shadow leaves the cadaver.
> During sleep, a splitting sometimes occurs, as indicated by dreams
> ... If one dreams of a deceased person, or an absent person, it is the
> shadow that appears to the sleeper. If a sick person's shadow tra-
> verses the dream of a parent living in another village, it is consid-
> ered a favorable sign that the sick person will recover ... A
> pregnant mother during a dream may see an ancestor who tells of
> his or her intention to be reborn in the body of the child. She offers
> a bit of cooked rice in thanks to the ancestor and as a request that
> the protection of the child not be withdrawn.[21]

In an older example, C. W. Hobley reports that for the Kamba
of East Africa, "a pregnant woman will sometimes dream of a deceased person night after night; if she dreams of a certain man
who is dead and then bears a son, they know it is that particular
man who has come back to earth, and the child will be given his
name."[22]

Despite the significance of dreams in many African cultures, I
would suggest that the incidence of birthmarks on repeater children (alleged to correspond to marks made on or possessed by a
deceased person) is so widely encountered in Africa that these

tangible manifestations should be given more credit for propagating the belief in reincarnation and the persistence in the spirit realm of deceased ancestors than the mere glimmerings from dreams or wishful yearnings for immortality. The importance of the repeater concept is demonstrated by the fact that it not only has been a passive belief but has led to active "experimentation"—the deliberate marking of cadavers for the express purpose of seeing if corresponding marks appeared on a subsequent child. We have emphasized the marking of the cadavers of deceased children, but the bodies of deceased adults are also marked. In his book on the Igbo, Victor C. Uchendu noted that he is alleged to be the reincarnation of an uncle.

> There is no doubt that my birth in 1930 relieved the anxiety of my parents. My name, Chikezie ("May God Create Well") is symbolic of what I meant to them. My family's confidence was doubled when the diviner returned his verdict that I was Ufomadu reincarnated. Ufomadu was my father's immediate older brother, the third of the four sons of my father's mother. On his deathbed, he had advised my father to marry quickly for "he was coming back to him." The diviner's verdict could not be doubted: I have "birthmarks" (three black spots on the right side of my belly) to vindicate it! It is claimed by my father that my "birthmarks" resulted from the marks made on Ufomadu *post mortem* for the purpose of vindicating his "personality" in the next cycle of life, which I now represent.[23]

The impressions made on the minds of indigenous peoples by alleged repeater children with identifying marks were likely to have been extremely powerful. Even in Asian cultures where ancestor worship and reincarnation constitute the main dogma of human existence, a belief in repeater children may have been decisive at some stage in implanting the belief. In Hindu circles, ancestor worship has been superseded by the pantheon of gods, but the principle of reincarnation is still widely accepted. Buddhism has similar features, since in certain respects Buddhism can be considered to have arisen as a Hindu reform movement. Therefore it is of special interest that a report by N. E. Parry from the Assam-Burma region of Southeast Asia describes marking practices on cadavers similar to those encountered in Africa.

> Although the Lakhers hold that when an adult dies the spirit goes to Athikhi, whence it never returns, there is a strong belief that the

spirits of children are sometimes reborn in the person of a younger brother or sister, and I have been given definite instances in support of this belief. In Longba village one Seikia and his wife Tleihia had a son called Laikha. To the great grief of his parents, Laikha died when he was about five years old. Before burying Laikha, his mother made a mark on his ankle with soot from off the cooking-pot, and when the corpse was laid in the grave the parents called out, "Come back to us again." After a while Tleihia gave birth to another son, on whose ankle is a black mark similar to that made on Laikha's ankle before he was buried. This boy was given the two names Laikha and Laribai, and is now about nine years old.[24]

Parry cites a number of other examples, and a similar practice has been reported recently in Thailand by I. Stevenson. In the case studied by Stevenson, the repeater child, Ampam Petcherat, possessed a birthmark on the chest alleged to correspond to a red ochre mark placed on the cadaver of a deceased child in a nearby village.[25]

These similar practices in Africa and Asia raise the possibility that the underlying beliefs were spread by migrations. Strong linguistic evidence exists for migrations from Borneo to Madagascar. Alternatively, the beliefs and practices could have arisen independently, following from precursor beliefs in reincarnation or as an effort to explain birth defects. If some unusual genetic abnormality was present in a population group that led, for example, to the absence of the last bone of the left little finger, then some accident of a deceased person that resulted in partial amputation of a finger could have been identified as a causal factor. Once the belief took hold, if more and more cadavers were marked, more opportunities for explaining various birthmarks would be available, and the belief would be solidified.

There are some difficulties with this line of argument. One difficulty is that the birthmarks are sometimes so irregular (different fingers affected on the left and right hands) that they depart from the concepts of teratology (the science of the study of abnormal formations of the body) derived from embryology. Another difficulty is that a lack of rigor must be assumed in "confusing" the locations or exact correspondence of marks on cadavers to birthmarks on children. However, the remarkable talents that led to achievements such as bronze casting in cultures with no written language imply powers of observation and retention not readily reconciled with a "confusion" of cadaver marks and birthmarks.

Whatever the true origin of the concept—pure fantasy, a historical consequence of sickle cell anemia, or some deep insight into the human condition—it is clear that the notion of repeater children, and the significance of the identifying marks they bear, have captured a position of prime importance in African mythology. The assertion by certain Igbo physicians that the *ogbanje* concept is the traditional identification of sickle cell anemia probably overstates the linkage, since the powers of traditional diagnosis are not likely to have been sufficiently reliable to yield a consistent interpretation. Nevertheless, the *ogbanje* concept and the finger-shortening ritual could well have historical origins in sickle cell anemia. The rituals of other African societies with a well developed mythology of repeater children are less obviously con-

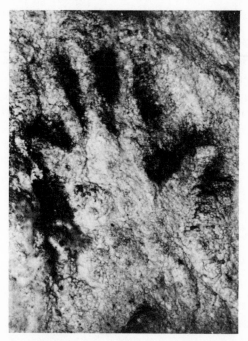

Figure 4.6. An imprint of a hand that appears to be missing the end of the left little finger from the Gargas grotto in the French Pyrenees Mountains. It bears a striking resemblance to the hands of the *ogbanje* children of Nigeria. Dating from prehistoric times, the walls of Gargas are covered with well over a hundred imprints of hands, the vast majority left hands, and nearly all missing some portion of one or more fingers. (From C. Barrière.)

nected to fingers and hence to sickling, but a great deal more research is needed to obtain a clearer overview. Deliberate mutilations may have played a number of different roles in the past, as far back as prehistoric times (Fig. 4.6), possibly including acceptance into certain secret societies and protection to render the individual unacceptable for slave commerce.[26] The marking of cadavers may have also served to warn the mother to restrain bonding if the next baby had the same sign, so as to limit the grief that would arise if the second child were also to leave prematurely.

In pursuing possible cultural implications of sickle cell anemia, we have thus been led into a consideration of a number of subtle issues of traditional African society. In such areas, conclusions are never as certain as for the structure of a helix or the sequence of bases in DNA, and definitive conclusions may never be achieved. Nevertheless, the repeater children are a fascinating topic for future anthropological research, although opportunities for such research may not be long-lived. As African societies move into the modern technological culture of our planet, the importance of repeater children is likely to wane, but sickle cell anemia will not be so easily eliminated. Therefore, the remaining topics to be presented concern efforts to deal with the effects of sickling through modern molecular biology and pharmacology.

CHAPTER 5

THE MOLECULAR PERSPECTIVE

While virtually every facet of traditional African life has been linked to mythology, in our scientifically oriented society it is molecules that have taken on mythic proportions. As one property after another of living organisms has been explained in molecular terms—including many aspects of genetic inheritance and cellular activity—the power of the scientific method looms as if without limit. Although we can readily recognize its successes, and delineate certain fundamental differences compared with the parallel science of traditional societies, the scientific method itself is not so easily characterized. Scientists carry out their research without explaining in abstract terms what it is they are doing. Molecules are isolated, properties are measured, experiments are formulated to permit mechanisms to be deduced, but with a wide variety of styles and strategies, depending on the nature of the problem at hand and the personal qualities of the scientist.

In an effort to describe the modern science that contrasts with the parallel science of traditional Africa, it is necessary to recognize this diversity of what we call modern science. Even for the relatively simple subject of hemoglobin, many examples of this diversity will be encountered. Hemoglobin has played a part in several major developments during the rise of molecular biology, and many leading scientists have given it their attention in ways that inevitably illustrate their particular styles and strategies. As a result, hemoglobin can serve us in three ways, providing: (1) the essential molecular ingredient needed to explain sickle cell disease; (2) a tool in helping to reveal how science and scientists function; and (3) a reference point for discussing the major processes of molecular biology.

The mythic role of molecules in our scientific society is especially apparent when we consider the impact of discoveries in molecular biology on our perception of the human condition. With its basis in experimental evidence and refutable hypotheses, the scientific method conveys the primacy of objective knowledge over any scientifically untestable orthodoxy. One consequence has been the erosion of the historical sense of "purpose" to life. Molecular biology has demonstrated that we are created according to the messages in the DNA of our genes. The strings of information in the four-letter alphabet of these messages are translated according to the rules of the genetic code into chains of amino acids with their twenty-letter alphabet. The amino acid sequences then spontaneously fold into highly ordered, three-dimensional proteins that carry out the various biochemical functions with remarkable efficiency. No protein designed by scientists working in the laboratory has come close to rivaling the efficiency of a natural protein.

All cells operate through the expression, in the form of proteins, of information transmitted by DNA, and all living things are organized in terms of cells. In the extreme view, the only imperative throughout evolution that even resembles an intrinsic purpose has been the need for DNA to replicate and to specify through the genes more efficient organisms in which to carry out its molecular act. Few biologists have tried to carry this molecular perspective to its philosophical limits; one who did was Jacques Monod, who reflected on the idea of objective knowledge and how it has permeated biology and beyond:

> Cold and austere, proposing no explanation but imposing an ascetic renunciation of all other spiritual fare, this idea was not of a kind to allay anxiety, but aggravated it instead. By a single stroke it claimed to sweep away the tradition of a hundred thousand years, which had become one with human nature itself. It wrote an end to the ancient animist covenant between man and nature, leaving nothing in place of that precious bond but an anxious quest in a frozen universe of solitude. With nothing to recommend it but a certain puritan arrogance, how could such an idea win acceptance?

It did not; it still has not. It has however commanded recognition; but that is because, solely because, of its prodigious power of performance.[1]

Not everyone would extend the molecular perspective as far as has Monod, nor give such a somber outlook if they did. Personally, I find the prospects of liberation from the old dogmas and the possibility of "reinventing" the human condition very invigorating and exciting, but whatever the prognosis, those who care to think about it can hardly deny that molecular biology is responsible for a revolution in our concepts of ourselves. The groundwork was laid by Darwin's insight into evolution—that natural selection will, when coupled with the inherent variations associated with reproduction of biological organisms, lead to the proliferation of organisms with the seeming, but only seeming, purpose of mastering their environment. Selection thus emerges as an effectively automatic process that will lead to the perpetuation of favorable characteristics. However, with no insight into the mechanisms of heredity, evolution in Darwin's terms remained a somewhat abstract concept. The possibility remained that a wholly new "vitalist" principle, a principle apart from conventional physics and chemistry, might still emerge to explain heredity. Then, with the unraveling of the intimate workings of genes in purely chemical terms, the new facts of life became inescapable.

Monod's attention to the philosophical implications of molecular biology came near the end of a highly productive career at the Pasteur Institute in Paris. His research contributed greatly to the understanding of how genes are organized in bacteria and how their expression is controlled. This interest in control mechanisms led eventually to his work on hemoglobin. Coupled with his achievements in science was his reputation in other spheres—as a leader of the French resistance during the war and as an outspoken activist in the Camus tradition. Every scientist is a composite of many individual tendencies, but a large part of Monod's success was due, I believe, to his particular qualities as a "strategist" in his approach to science. The strategist puts the emphasis on formulating theories and subsequently designing experiments to test them. This approach contrasts with the style of a "phenomenologist"—the scientist who studies a process and is led by the results into more and more detailed studies, with the results of one study leading the investigation into the next. Various approaches are valuable in science, as I will try to show, and the same scientist may employ varied approaches at different times, in response to different problems. Labels are therefore always somewhat arbitrary and exaggerated. Nevertheless, Monod's career is a useful illustration, because he deliberately tried to carry his reasoning as far as possible, into both the social consequences of biological beliefs and the action of proteins and the properties of hemoglobin.

One of Monod's last major papers, with Jeffries Wyman and Jean-Pierre Changeux, proposed a new way of understanding a perplexing aspect of oxygen binding by hemoglobin that had first attracted the attention of scientists at the beginning of the century.[2] Hemoglobin had long played a central role in biochemistry, since it is readily identifiable because of its striking red color and is easily isolated from red blood cells (which are effectively little bags of nearly pure hemoglobin). When oxygen binding to hemoglobin was studied in detail, it was found that the binding of a small amount of oxygen promoted the binding of additional oxygen. This "cooperativity" was the intriguing process that Monod set out to explain. However, before discussing cooperativity and the explanation presented by Monod and his colleagues, we should note that what placed hemoglobin firmly in the limelight of molecular biology was its role in the formation of sickled cells. In 1949 Linus Pauling and his research team made a key observation concerning sickle cell anemia that was a landmark as well in the history of molecular biology.

Studying the migration of hemoglobin in electric fields, Pauling and his colleagues noted that sickled cells contain an altered form of hemoglobin that migrates less rapidly than the usual form. From this observation, the alteration in the overall shape of red blood cells was traced to the modification of just one protein. The altered form of this protein was called hemoglobin S, and sickle cell anemia was designated a "molecular disease." The migration of hemoglobin in an electric field, a technique called electrophoresis, is still one of the tools used to identify hemoglobin S. Linus Pauling also made a number of other major contributions to hemoglobin research, including one of the early explanations of cooperativity.[3]

Several years after sickling was related to molecules, another dramatic development placed the understanding of sickling at the level of an "atomic disease." Vernon Ingram demonstrated that the only alteration in hemoglobin S was in just one of the amino acids found in hemoglobin's beta chains.[4] As noted in Chapter 2, hemoglobin is composed of four separate parts, called subunits or chains: two alpha chains, each made up of a sequence of 141 amino acids, and two beta chains, each made up of a sequence of 146 amino acids. Although the alpha chains are slightly shorter than the beta chains, both are very similar in overall structure. In hemoglobin S the amino acid normally at the sixth position of the beta chains, glutamic acid, is replaced by a different amino acid, valine. Glutamic acid is a charged amino acid that is very soluble in water, whereas valine is an uncharged amino acid that is poorly soluble in water. The loss of charge explained the original observation by Pauling and his colleagues of slower migration in an electric field. In addition, it seemed plausible, and has since been confirmed, that the uncharged, poorly soluble valine residues create a sticky spot that causes the hemoglobin molecules to adhere to one another and form elongated structures that distort the red cells into their characteristic sickle shape.

The more immediate impact of hemoglobin S on molecular biology was to dramatize the fact that information in genes must be of a sufficiently discrete form to specify individual amino acids. Biochemists were beginning to appreciate that every organism contains thousands of different proteins, each made up of a defined sequence of amino acids. These individual proteins each serve an important function—some as enzymes catalyzing one of the myriad reactions of cellular metabolism, others with roles in cell structure and movement (such as muscle proteins), transport (such as hemoglobin), or recognition (such as hormone receptors). The sizes of proteins range from scores to hundreds of amino acids, and all proteins are built from a set of just twenty different kinds of amino acids. Somehow the information for specifying the amino acid sequences of all of these proteins is stored in the genes of the chromosomes. Each protein is specified by a different gene, but in the 1950s biochemists could not yet explain how the information stored in the gene was translated into the sequence of amino acids for the corresponding proteins. Thus, the discovery that just one amino acid is changed in hemoglobin S demonstrated that, whatever the mechanism of gene translation, it must work amino acid by amino acid, rather than in fixed groups of amino acids.

The stage had been set some years earlier for beginning to explain the action of genes, when James Watson and Francis Crick electrified the scientific world with their description of the structure of the molecules of genes, deoxyribonucleic acid or DNA, in terms of the remarkable double helix.[5] The structure appeared as two strands of nucleotide bases in an almost endless spiral staircase. The long strands were made up of a particular sequence of four chemically distinct bases, adenine, thymine, guanine, and cytosine (abbreviated as A, T, G, and C), with each "step" of the spiral staircase formed by a pair of bases, either A paired with T or G paired with C. In a single stoke, the double helix revealed how DNA was built of strands linked by base pairs (thereby explaining why the amounts of A and T are equal, as are the amounts of G and C, in the DNA from various species), and proposed a method for the conservation of genetic information during cell division by replication of DNA. Every time a cell divides, the two strands separate and the "missing" strand in each daughter cell is replaced by a new strand whose sequence of bases is determined by the A-with-T and G-with-C pairing. Thus each "old" strand provides a template for the "new" strand, producing two molecules of DNA from one. In this way the genetic heritage of a cell is maintained in both of the two new cells, each of which contains DNA molecules made up of one strand from the parent cell and one newly synthesized strand.

This scheme also permitted the first understanding of evolution at the molecular level. By dividing to form germ cells (a process called meiosis), cells can pass their DNA on to subsequent generations. Random changes in the sequence of bases (mutations) in the germ lines would automatically be incorporated into the offspring, so that new or altered genes that lead to improved proteins would be perpetuated in the march of evolution.

More than any other discovery in molecular biology, DNA typifies the mythic aspect of molecules in our society, as the double helix is a powerful vehicle for evolution worthy of any deity. The discovery of the DNA double helix remains one of the most interesting moments in the history of molecular biology and justifies the attention that it has been given by scientists and historians. As with most events in science, however, the situation is never as simple as it appears at first glance. It has subsequently been discovered that genetic information can be stored in other molecules (the RNA of certain viruses, including many of the viruses implicated in cancer) and that DNA can apparently exist in other very different helical forms (the left-handed helix known as Z-DNA that is distinct from the original right-handed helix proposed by Watson and Crick).[6]

After the identification of the double helix, the next frontier was to discover the details of the genetic code by which combinations of the four nucleotide bases that make up the genes of DNA specify the sequences of amino acids in proteins. The sequence of bases in a gene is first transcribed into many copies of another type of nucleic acid, messenger ribonucleic acid, or mRNA, and the mRNA sequence of bases is translated into the corresponding sequence of amino acids on specialized particles called ribosomes. In the decade following the discovery of the double helix, methods using artificial mRNA molecules were developed which permitted the genetic code to be deduced. These methods established that a triplet of three bases specifies each of the 20 amino acids. There are 64 unique triplets, or codons, but in most cases a single amino acid can be specified by several different codons, particularly sets differing in the third position.

When the amino acids corresponding to each codon were determined, it then became apparent that a change in a single base of the DNA in the three-base codon for glutamic acid (GAG) would convert it to the codon for valine (GTG). Thus, sickling was traced to a single base change (A to T) in the DNA of the beta-globin gene.

Formally, the system for storing information in genes is arbitrary. Since each position in the DNA is occupied by one of four bases, we can represent each position in computer notation with two bits:

$$A: 11 \qquad G: 10$$
$$T: 00 \qquad C: 01$$

Thus, with two characters, 0 and 1, it is possible to describe four combinations to represent the four bases A, T, G, and C. Moreover, if we assume that in the double helix pairing takes place only between the forms 0 and 1, then only the pairs A-T and G-C will be permitted. Therefore, from the point of view of information theory, the genetic information can be readily represented by this simple notation, and each amino acid can be defined by codons of three units of double bits; for example, the GTG codon for valine becomes 100010. In essence, the storage of a text in a computer works in the same way, using eight bits for each letter, although depending on whether the computer is from IBM or Apple, the same letters can have different representation in the computer, since different encoding patterns are used.

For life on earth, amino acids always have the same representation in the DNA (with the exception of the representation of several amino acids in subcellular structures known as mitochondria), but we have no reason to reject the idea that some other representation with its corresponding genetic code would do just as well, in analogy with the different coding patterns of Apple and IBM computers. For example, we can provide no arguments why exchange of A with G and T with C, with the corresponding changes in the genetic code, would not work as well as the existing system. It is in this respect that the genetic code appears to be arbitrary regarding the actual assignments of amino acids to codons. However, when we come to the 20-letter alphabet of the amino acids in proteins, a different principle applies, since the amino acids are not fulfilling a symbolic function but a structural one. Therefore, the proper analogy is not with computer representation, or even with English, which is also a symbolic language. Rather, the amino acids are more analogous to a language with characters like Chinese or hieroglyphics. Each amino acid has a shape and a structure that has a particular meaning in chemical terms (size, charge, reactivity, and so on) and therefore is not at all arbitrary, but corresponds to some precise chemical function. While many mutations have little or no effect on proteins (because these mutations produce an alternate codon for the same amino acid or the codon for an amino acid with properties similar to the original amino acid), in some cases changing one of these amino acid "characters" can greatly alter the properties of the protein—precisely the consequence of the replacement of a glutamic acid by valine in hemoglobin S.

We shall return in Chapter 7 to the base change in DNA responsible for forming the sickle variant of hemoglobin, since it is at the core of new methods used to diagnose sickle cell anemia in fetuses. Treatment of sicklers at the level of their DNA is a possible antisickling measure that we shall also consider. However, most of the activity in the field of sickle cell research since the pivotal observations of Pauling and his colleagues and Ingram has been directed toward hemoglobin. In order to understand the molecular mechanism of sickling and in order to design possible chemical modifications of hemoglobin able to block sickling, all aspects of the properties of hemoglobin S have been intensely scrutinized. Since the characteristics of oxygen binding by hemoglobin are intimately related to the sickling process, we will now explore oxygen binding and describe efforts of Monod and Pauling to clarify the process.

Hemoglobin molecules within red blood cells bind oxygen tightly as the cells pass through the capillaries of the lungs. As the red cells circulate through the heart and on to the muscles and other organs that require oxygen, the hemoglobin loosens its hold so that the oxygen can pass readily out of the red cells and into the tissues where it is needed. Thus, the structure of hemoglobin somehow evolved to modulate or regulate its own binding of oxygen. This feature of a "molecular servo-mechanism," or more simply "cooperativity" between the oxygen binding sites, has attracted great interest among several generations of biochemists. The cooperativity was recognized initially in terms of a "sigmoidal" or S-shaped curve for the description of the binding of oxygen by hemoglobin. The more usual "noncooperative" binding reaction is characterized by a simpler "hyperbolic" curve that implies an unchanging binding strength. Therefore, the sigmoidal curve reveals a much more complicated process in which some binding favors more binding (as would occur in the lungs), or, considered from the opposite perspective, some release favors more release (as would occur in the muscles).

The cooperativity reflected by the S-shaped curve suggests a level of communication between different oxygen binding events more commonly associated with animate objects or people. It is easy to find analogies to the S-shaped curve in everyday experience. For example, at the community swimming pool, a typical day has something in common with oxygen binding by hemoglobin. The first to arrive do not all go immediately into the pool— the temperature is not yet at its peak and the water looks cold, so a graph of the occupancy of the pool as a function of the number of people present would have a shallow slope. As the day proceeds, the population around the pool rises and more and more people enter the pool—seemingly enticed to enter by the sight of other swimmers—and the slope of the graph rises. Eventually the pool becomes very crowded, and as more people arrive they cannot all fit into the pool, consequently, the slope of the graph levels off, with occupancy of the pool approaching saturation. Overall, the process fits nicely to an S-shaped curve. In contrast, if we monitor the limited number of chairs around the pool, we see that their occupancy rises steeply with the increasing population and saturates at a relatively low population, following a simple saturation process typified by a hyperbolic curve.

The advantage of the cooperativity of hemoglobin is dramatized by comparing its behavior with a simple hyperbolic system, such as the oxygen-binding protein myoglobin found in muscle (Fig. 5.1). In concert with the evolution of hemoglobin in blood cells, myoglobin developed to bind oxygen in muscles. If we mark with arrows the points on the figure that correspond to the oxygen concentrations in lungs and muscles, we see that cooperativity permits a very efficient release of oxygen into the muscles after

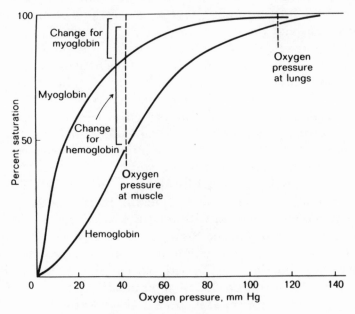

Figure 5.1. The oxygen-binding curves for hemoglobin and myoglobin.

full saturation in the lungs. In contrast, if hemoglobin followed the pattern given by the hyperbolic curve, a much smaller fraction of the oxygen it had bound in the lungs would be available for release in the muscles. Myoglobin, because it follows the hyperbolic curve, can in fact bind the oxygen released by the hemoglobin to facilitate its uptake in the muscles. Since individual muscles will eventually use up all of their oxygen, such low levels of oxygen will be reached that the myoglobin will then release the oxygen it has bound. Thus, from a functional point of view, it is easy to see why the S-shaped binding curve of hemoglobin presented a great evolutionary advantage, since it permits such efficient oxygen delivery. We can also begin to appreciate why scientists have long been fascinated with trying to understand how hemoglobin achieves its cooperative interactions.

The framework for explaining the mechanism of hemoglobin's cooperativity was narrowed considerably in the 1920s, when precise measurements indicated that each molecule of hemoglobin binds four molecules of oxygen. The binding of each oxygen (in the diatomic form, O_2) takes place at an iron atom at the center of a complex ring structure called a heme. Thus, the two alpha and the two beta subunits of hemoglobin each have a heme embedded in their structure. Although the name hemoglobin was selected originally for other reasons, we can think of it as representing the combination of "heme" and "globin." The specific changes in the tightness of oxygen binding by hemoglobin in different parts of the body, which we have characterized as cooperativity or "communication" between oxygen binding sites, came to be called the "heme–heme interactions."

One of the early efforts to explain the basis of the heme–heme interactions was made in 1935 by Linus Pauling. Little was known about the detailed structure of hemoglobin at the time, and Pauling imagined that the hemes were in close or near contact, such that binding of oxygen at one heme could have a direct effect on the neighboring hemes. He recognized that interesting patterns in the possible combinations of hemoglobin with oxygen arose from the fact that hemoglobin has four oxygen-binding sites. His model was presented in precise mathematical terms, but in its essentials the model has game-like qualities that could be used to illustrate the principles of the model. We can call the game "hold your hats."

If we imagine four New World monkeys at the corners of a square, we can picture them facing the center of the square surrounded by hats. At various times, one or more of the monkeys will put on a hat. When a monkey is wearing a hat, he can also help to hold the hat on the head of each of the other monkeys of his quartet wearing a hat, but monkeys without hats cannot hold the hats of others. Thus, when all of the monkeys are wearing hats, each can help to hold on the hats of the other three (which is why the game requires New World monkeys, since they have two hands and a tail to place on the heads of the other monkeys to hold their hats). Now we imagine that a hat buyer comes along. The price of a hat is set at $1 for each monkey wearing or holding the hat. If only one monkey has a hat on, no others are available to help hold it on and the price is simply $1. However, when two monkeys are wearing hats, each can help to hold the other's and the price of each hat becomes $2. When three monkeys are wearing hats, each can hold the hats of the other two and the price of each hat becomes $3. Finally, when all monkeys are hatted, each hat will be held by three others and the price will be $4. In this way we have created a game in which the price of hats increases systematically with the number of hats worn.

If we consider the price a reflection of how tightly the monkeys are holding on to their hats, then we arrive at a situation close to the properties of oxygen binding by hemoglobin—the more hats (or oxygen) present, the tighter each is bound, as the tightness is reinforced by the interactions between several players or units. In the Pauling model it is the hemes that are at the corners of a square, and the interactions between hemes with oxygens bound are assumed to provide the stabilizing interactions which cause the oxygens to be bound more tightly in the same manner that the interactions in our game caused the price of the hats to rise. In molecular terms, the interactions between heme units have, of course, certain distinct chemical features, but the principle of sequentially increasing strength of oxygen binding is formally identical to those in the game. Thus, for the Pauling model, oxygen binding is cooperative, because each step of oxygen binding permits more stabilizing interactions—none with the first, 1 with the second, 2 with the third, and 3 with the fourth—in the same pattern as the price of the hats. As a result, this simple geometric model explained, at least in principle, how the heme–heme inter-actions might arise.

Pauling proposed his model at a time when only a few details about the structure of hemoglobin were known. When the complete three-dimensional structure of hemoglobin was later solved by x-ray diffraction from its crystals, the hemes were found to be a considerable distance apart (Fig. 5.2). Therefore, the heme–heme interactions could not occur by direct contact, but the Pauling model could still apply with the intervention of indirect contacts transmitted through the protein structure. Indeed, as testimony to its ingenuity, more than 30 years after its formulation this same scheme served as the basis for a modernized version championed by Daniel Koshland and his colleagues. Their ideas were built around the concept of "induced fit" whereby binding of small

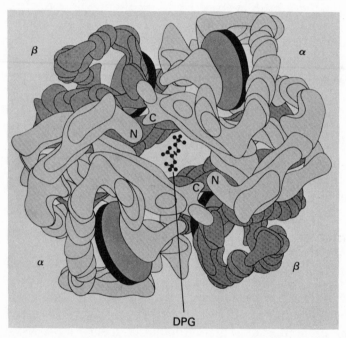

Figure 5.2. The three-dimensional structure of hemoglobin as determined by x-ray crystallography in the laboratory of Max Perutz. The location of the binding site for DPG in the central cavity between the beta chains is shown. The disklike objects represent the hemes. (Adapted from Perutz, "The hemo-globin molecule." Copyright © 1964 by Scientific American, Inc. All rights reserved.)

molecules like oxygen to proteins could "instruct" or "direct" the proteins to take the correct shape to bind the small molecules tightly. In this view, as each chain bound oxygen, a change in structure was induced that enhanced the binding to other sub-units. Therefore, the strength of binding would rise progressively as oxygen was bound, with precisely the same mathematical basis as the Pauling model or our game with hats.[7]

Ideas similar to Pauling's original "instructive" mechanism were in vogue at the time also to explain the existence of a vast array of different antibodies in each individual capable of bind-ing to a seemingly unlimited number of antigens. Pauling and others had proposed that the antigen "instructs" the antibody to assume the correct shape needed to bind the antigen. In a formal sense these ideas are somewhat analogous to the pre-Darwinian idea that the giraffe evolved from ancestors who stretched their necks reaching for higher and higher branches and then passed their elongated necks on to their descendants. We, of course, now see this view as flawed, since there is no mechanism for transmit-ting the acquired characteristics. The key to Darwinian evolution is the spontaneous appearance of characteristics such as long necks, independent of their usefulness. A longer neck arises by random variation in the genes, but the survival (and reproduc-tive) advantage it confers leads to its perpetuation in the pop-ulation. For hemoglobin, in contrast to Pauling's basically instructive idea, it was the development of a "selection" principle by Monod and his collaborators that revolutionized thinking about these problems. The key element was the prior existence of minor conformations of hemoglobin, that is, molecules with the same chemical structure but with slightly different positions of the atoms due to rotations of chemical bonds. Certain such con-formations were postulated to possess the capacity to bind oxygen tightly. When oxygen was present, such minor forms would be preferentially stabilized by oxygen, or in effect "selected," and become predominant. The mathematics of such a process fits the oxygen binding just as well as the Pauling sequential binding. However, in order to reach this detailed description of this pro-cess, Monod had first considered several other aspects of the problem.

Monod and his colleagues argued that at an early stage of evo-lution hemoglobin subunits were already likely to have achieved the capacity for binding oxygen very efficiently. Therefore, they concluded, it was unlikely that the association of the hemoglobin subunits could provide a boost to oxygen binding through stronger interactions between oxygenated subunits. Rather, they reasoned that any changes associated with interactions between subunits were likely to decrease the tightness of oxygen binding. Hence, a key feature of Monod's model was an antagonism between the binding of oxygen and the mutual binding between unoxygenated subunits. This view agrees with the finding that when hemoglobin is taken apart, the isolated subunits do indeed bind oxygen very tightly. On these grounds alone Pauling's model for heme–heme interactions cannot be correct as originally formulated, but it could be revised to incorporate this feature.

For example, in our game of hats, we could assume that each monkey places his hand or tail on the head of another monkey only when both are hatless. If we then imagine the arrival of a hat distributor, we can stipulate that he pay $1 to each monkey to wear a hat, plus $1 to each monkey who must remove his hand or tail for the hat to be worn. Then the first hat will cost the distributor $4, the second $3, the third $2, and the last will cost only $1. Thus, the effort or cost of putting on the hats diminishes as more hats are added, just as the binding of oxygen by hemoglobin in the lungs is facilitated as more is bound. We have simply changed the monkeys' interactions from positive or enhancing (holding the hats on) to negative or constraining (blocking the wearing of hats). Either model can in principle represent equally well the cooperative binding of oxygen by hemoglobin, but the negative type of interaction is more likely for the reasons cited.

A second argument advanced by Monod was that when subunits associate to form multisubunit proteins, as in the case of the four subunits of hemoglobin, certain kinds of symmetry occur which would be maintained throughout various stages of oxygenation. The principal type of symmetry involves a twofold rotational axis (also called a dyad axis). In this form of symmetry, one object can be superimposed on its symmetrically related partner by a rotation of 180 degrees about the twofold axis. Roughly speaking, this form of symmetry resembles an "embrace," in which the two objects contribute corresponding surfaces to the contact, as in the Brancusi sculpture "The Kiss" (Fig. 5.3), although to be strictly correct for twofold symmetry the two part-

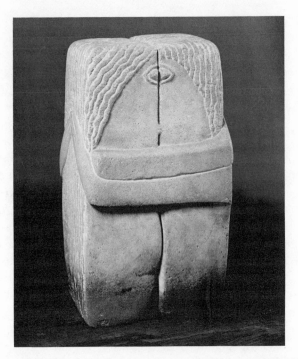

Figure 5.3. "The Kiss" by Constantin Brancusi. The two figures have near, but not perfect, symmetry. (From the Louise and Walter Arensberg Collection of the Philadelphia Museum of Art. Photographed by Eric Mitchell, 1984.)

ners should be identical twins. The alternate arrangement, as in objects lined up "front to back" or "head to tail," would place different surfaces at the contact between any two of the objects. Monod called the embrace arrangement "isologous association," to indicate that the subunits contribute identical surface areas to the contact, whereas the alternative arrangement was designated "heterologous association." As Jean-Pierre Changeux, a coauthor of the classic 1965 paper, recalls,

> For either esthetic or (more likely) practical reasons, Jacques Monod always preferred the isologous association. It . . . automatically confers a twofold axis of symmetry and thus oligomers built by isologous association possess more symmetry properties than those of heterologous association. They always have even numbers of subunits, which explains Jacques Monod's quasi-mystical opposition to trimers and pentamers.[8]

Hemoglobin is indeed constructed along isologous lines, with the alpha and beta subunits related by a pseudo-twofold axis (pseudo, since the two kinds of subunits are similar but not identical, as the partners in "The Kiss") to form a dimer. Then two dimers associate with a true twofold axis to complete the hemoglobin tetramer. It can be demonstrated that the association of four subunits to give a tetramer is the largest number of subunits that a protein based entirely on twofold symmetry can have and remain a "closed" or "self-limited" structure. If tetramers themselves associate with twofold axes, the identical bonding surfaces would be available on opposite sides of the tetramers, and "open" or "unlimited" structures, such as crystals or long chains of molecules, would result. For example, considering again "The Kiss," two identical versions of the sculpture could be connected at their respective bases to form a "tetramer" analogous to hemoglobin. However, if copies of these tetramers were to be connected again, say at their heads, infinite chains of tetramers would result, since each tetramer would have heads at opposite ends. In this way we see that the tetramer has special qualities that cannot be found, for example, in an octamer. As a consequence, it seemed to Monod no mere coincidence that hemoglobin and many other proteins were composed of four subunits.

The final step in Monod's thinking concerned the mechanism of cooperativity between oxygen binding sites. He assumed that the sites were not in direct contact and must cooperate by some "allosteric" mechanism. He coined the word "allosteric" from its Greek roots, meaning different sites or different structures. This word has come to be widely used in describing the various interactions found in proteins possessing properties of cooperativity. Since Monod believed that symmetry would be preserved throughout oxygen binding, he was led to postulate the existence of different forms with slightly different shapes. The studies of protein structure in crystals tended to give static representations, as if interactions between the amino acids within a protein were frozen like the bricks in a building. In reality, protein structure is constantly in motion, with the detailed positions of each amino acid continuously changing by small amounts as the overall structure fluctuates about its most stable conformations. Different forms rapidly interconvert; for hemoglobin, conformations with different potential strengths for binding oxygen would be present even in the absence of oxygen. Forms of a protein having the same chemical structure but slightly varying shapes are known as "conformational states."

Monod and his colleagues postulated that in the absence of oxygen there would be a principal conformational state for hemoglobin characterized by strong interactions between its subunits but only a weak capacity to bind oxygen. This state was designated "T" for the tight interactions between the subunits. In the absence of oxygen, the vast majority of the population of molecules would be in the T state. However, another state was also postulated, characterized by weaker interactions between its subunits but the capacity to bind oxygen tightly. This state was designated "R" for the relaxed interactions between the subunits. In the absence of oxygen, only a miniscule fraction of the population of hemoglobin molecules would be in the R state. However, if the hemoglobin molecules were in the presence of oxygen, the oxygen would bind preferentially to the R-state molecules and they would become more stable owing to the oxygen binding. In this way the oxygen would "select" the R state, and as more and more oxygen was added, a larger and larger fraction of the molecules would be stabilized in the R state. When oxygen saturation reached 100%, the R state would be the majority state, with the T state represented by only a small fraction of the population. Thus, oxygenation would cause a transition from a population of hemoglobin molecules dominated by the T state to a population dominated by the R state. The transition is always concerted, such that symmetry is conserved in passing between the T and R states, with no molecules composed of an intermediate mixture of subunits in T and R.

To grasp the concept of preexisting conformational states, we can imagine another version of our game with New World monkeys. In this case, since the essential concept is a distribution of molecules between the T and R states, we need to imagine thousands of monkeys in sets of four. As in the case of the "negative" formulation of the Pauling model, each monkey will initially have its hands and tail on the heads of its three partners, thereby interfering with their wearing a hat. Since all the monkeys perform the same gesture of covering their neighbors' heads, each group (which we can designate T) exhibits "symmetry." We must next imagine that occasionally a set of four monkeys all remove their hands and tails from their partners' heads in concert to produce a band of four with exposed heads. Thus, the four monkeys in a group with exposed heads (which we can designate R) will also exhibit "symmetry." For the bareheaded monkeys, after a short time in this arrangement, they will, again in concert, recover one another's heads. However, elsewhere in the population of groups, others will from time to time bare their heads in concert.

We should now imagine that every time a set of monkeys becomes bareheaded, a hat distributor will place hats on their heads. Once hatted, the monkeys are less likely to cover their heads with their hands and tail. As more and more hats are available, more and more sets of monkeys will have their heads covered, until at "saturation" the vast majority of monkeys at any time will be hatted and only a tiny fraction will be hatless. The swing in population to the R arrangement is thus stabilized or "selected" by the hats. This game is a reasonable analogy for oxygen binding by hemoglobin according to the model of T and R states. In the absence of oxygen the population is mainly in the T state but swings to the R state as oxygen is added, thereby converting most of the population into the form that binds oxygen strongly. Although somewhat complicated in execution, the model of R and T states is extremely simple in its formulation.

Initially Monod's concept of "selection" by oxygen from a preexisting mixture of symmetrical conformations was contrary to much of the "instructive" thinking of the time, and his model met with considerable skepticism, particularly by established investigators involved with hemoglobin research. Although distinct conformations had previously been identified from studies of crystals of deoxyhemoglobin and oxyhemoglobin by Max Perutz and his colleagues, most scientists imagined a gradual transition between the two forms, as oxygen was bound, involving a series of intermediate states. Monod emphasized that the differences between deoxyhemoglobin (identified with the T state) and oxyhemoglobin (identified with the R state) were sufficient to explain cooperativity without intermediate states. The difference included an increased spacing between the beta chains in the T state that creates a pocket for the binding of the small molecule 2,3-diphosphoglycerate (abbreviated DPG), as indicated in Figure 5.2. The binding of DPG contributes to the stability of the T state relative to the R state, since in the R state the beta chains move together and the DPG is expelled. Many other differences were also noted, but it was not obvious how the transition from one state to the other occurred. Currently, the arguments are at an extremely detailed level of molecular structure that would require an entire book to treat justly (indeed, several have already been written). Nevertheless, the principles presented here remain valid distinctions for the different explanations of cooperativity in oxygen binding by hemoglobin. To a large extent, Monod's theory has prevailed and has become the predominant way of looking at hemoglobin, since—as with every good theory—it predicted results that were not necessarily anticipated at the time the theory was formulated.

One such set of results that has especially interested me concerns the altered oxygen-binding properties of a number of genetic variants of hemoglobin. Following the discovery of hemoglobin S, many human population groups were screened by electrophoresis to identify hemoglobin S carriers. In the process, hemoglobin variants were detected that had neither the properties of normal adult hemoglobin (hemoglobin A) nor of hemoglobin S. In a short time many new hemoglobins were found and were initially designated with other letters of the alphabet. However, it soon became obvious that there were not going to be enough letters, and so the practice was changed to naming the hemoglobin after the geographical location of the discovery. Hundreds of such hemoglobin variants are now known, with the vast majority involving a change in just one amino acid at a particular position of either the alpha or beta chains. Their names range from cities of North America (such as hemoglobins Indianapolis, Detroit, and Ottawa) to more distant locations (such as hemoglobins Anantharaj, Hirosakim, Fort de France, Sherwood Forest, and Korle-Bu). In a number of cases, the hemoglobin variants possess strikingly abnormal oxygen-binding properties, with most (such as hemoglobin Chesapeake) binding oxygen much more tightly than hemoglobin A and a few (such as hemoglobin Kansas) binding oxygen much less tightly.

A confusing aspect about such variants was that both types— extra tight and extra loose oxygen binders—had very little cooperativity. When the first molecule of oxygen was lost from the fully oxygenated form, the remaining molecules of oxygen were still held almost as tightly as the first. I have been able to demonstrate that the behavior of both types of hemoglobin oxygen-binding variants could be explained by an alteration in the strength of the interactions between subunits that changed the preexisting distribution between the T and R states. For the extra-tight binder (hemoglobin Chesapeake), a large fraction of the molecules were in the R state even in the absence of oxygen. For the extra-loose oxygen binder (hemoglobin Kansas), the T state was over-stabilized, so that even after the binding of oxygen the molecules remained largely in the T state. For both types, the full allosteric T-to-R transition could not take place and as a result cooperativity was effectively lost.

The game with sets of monkeys can be used to describe the properties of the mutants if we assume that a hat can be placed loosely on the head of a T-state monkey even when it is covered with a hand or tail. The Monod model of R and T states thus easily accommodates the properties of mutant hemoglobins, whereas the sequential models of the Pauling type do not predict such changes in cooperativity. For this reason, studies of mutant hemoglobins have been among the major reasons for the general acceptance of the model of R and T states.

The same line of reasoning explains why the acidification of blood inhibits the binding of oxygen. This inhibition has important physiological consequences, since the active tissues such as muscle produce acids which liberate protons. When the oxygenated hemoglobin encounters these tissues, release of oxygen is stimulated beyond the level due to the heme–heme interactions. The stimulation of oxygen release caused by acid is known as the Bohr effect, named for its discoverer, Christian Bohr, father of the famous physicist Niels Bohr. The two-state model explains the Bohr effect by having the T state bind the protons liberated by acid more strongly than does the R state, thereby pushing the T-to-R transition in favor of the T state. However, in this case the change in the T-to-R equilibrium is not as drastic as for the mutant hemoglobins Chesapeake or Kansas, and cooperativity remains high.[9]

Other investigators studying rates of oxygen binding demonstrated that the model of T and R states could also be used readily to explain their results. At the present time, the T and R state formulation has been almost universally adopted by investigators of hemoglobin, at least in its broad outlines. Still, the casual usage of the terms has become so familiar that Monod's fundamental selection principle underlying the transition from the T to R state is often forgotten. As a result, even while discussing the T and R states, some investigators still speak of a "trigger" for the conformational change, and in so doing they return instinctively to the instructive formulation that the model of R and T states eliminates.

While a number of issues concerning the dynamics of the allosteric transition remain to be settled, the significance for sickled cells is clear. It is predominantly the molecules of hemoglobin S in the T state that associate with themselves to form fibers that distort red cells into the sickle shape. The association of the deoxygenated form of hemoglobin S is a key factor, as will be described in the next chapter, in explaining why sickling is found in regions where malaria is prevalent. In addition, changes in the T-to-R transition induced by possible antisickling agents that react with hemoglobin S are among the treatments for sickle cell anemia that we will consider in Chapter 8.

Although Pauling and Monod worked at different times and with different bases of data, two fundamentally different ways of thinking about the problem of cooperativity for hemoglobin are apparent in their approaches. Pauling represents the ingenious chemist. His most spectacular achievement was predicting the major pattern in the three-dimensional folding of chains of amino acids, a spring-like spiral known as the alpha helix. After Pauling's prediction, crystallographers who were working on the structures of myoglobin and hemoglobin confirmed that each subunit of hemoglobin is made up of eight interconnected stretches of alpha helix.

Undoubtedly, Pauling's deduction of the alpha helix was an incomparable tour-de-force. Moreover, as discussed in Chapter 2, he also pioneered in the use of hemoglobin from different species to measure the relative ages of species; this concept of a "biological clock" has had important consequences for understanding evolution. But when Pauling attempted to predict a model for DNA, his chemist's approach, based solely on chemical principles, broke down with his proposal of a three-stranded or triple helix. The double helix of Watson and Crick succeeded because of its reliance on biological principles. Not only did it fit the existing data, by postulating complementary base pairing of A with T and G with C, but it immediately suggested a mechanism for DNA replication by a parting of the two strands and a filling in of the missing strand by complementary base pairing. Here the biological perspective of Watson and Crick was critical.[10]

In another field, Pauling spent many years advancing an "instructive" model for antibody formation which relied on the antigen to induce the correct conformation. Antibody formation was later discovered to be a selection rather than an instruction process. We now know that when the body is confronted with a foreign substance (the antigen), it soon begins producing antibodies that specifically bind the antigen. These antibodies arise from antibody-producing cells, which employ a number of special mechanisms that spontaneously lead to recombination of genes for different portions of the antibody molecules. In this way an enormous population of cells is created, each of which produces one unique form of antibodies. The antigen binds with the cells that have the appropriate antibodies and stimulates their division and maturation into stable antibody-producing cells. Thus, the appropriate antibody-producing cells are "selected" by the antigen.

The point of reviewing these successes and failures is to show that certain types of thinking work best on certain problems. The intellectual qualities of Pauling and Monod serve to illustrate two types of virtuosity found in contemporary approaches to science: (1) deductions from precise measurements, as in Pauling's use of chemical information to arrive at the alpha helix; and (2) formulation of testable hypotheses by more intuitive approaches, as in Monod's model for hemoglobin. These distinctions for the two approaches are only approximate, as Pauling's achievements had elements of induction and Monod's had foundations in measurements, but taken together they form a fairly complete image of the principles that underlie modern science.

While Monod's approach was suitable for the problem of the cooperativity of oxygen binding by hemoglobin, in general it may have suffered from the weakness of being overly aesthetic. Monod himself once said, "A beautiful theory or model may not be right; but an ugly one must be wrong."[11] Yet the beauty of genes has recently been found to be marred by "messy" sequences of DNA called introns. Introns lie within genes but do not code for proteins; the alpha and beta globin genes each have two such introns. In the case of the globin genes, the regions interrupted by introns may represent archaic functions (such as heme binding or alpha–beta interaction) that were once associated with separate proteins. However, for many other proteins, the introns have no apparent purpose. Someone with Monod's aesthetic sense might have been predisposed against following the early leads that led to the discovery of introns. Clearly no single strategy presents the right approach for all circumstances.

The description of alternative modern approaches to science helps to place the parallel science practiced by traditional societies in a context that emphasizes acceptance of diversity. There is sufficient latitude in the strategies of modern scientists that we should be able to admit ideas from traditional approaches, although extracting reliable information may not be easy. We have already encountered some of the difficulties inherent in drawing conclusions when mythic concepts are involved, as in the question of the link between *ogbanje* and sickle cell anemia. A similar problem will be faced in exploring possible traditional medicines for use as antisickling agents (see Chapter 8). Ultimately, the modern and the mythic must be reconciled, if sickle cell anemia is to be successfully confronted in its African setting. In a reciprocal sense, lessons from studies of the dietary influences or traditional medicines from Africa may have an impact in improving the conditions of individuals with sickle cell anemia in the United States and other medically advanced countries.

CHAPTER 6

THE SICKLE HELIX

The bridge between sickle cell anemia, with its ramifications for individuals and societies, and the molecular world of DNA and hemoglobin is a surprising and awesome entity—the fibers of hemoglobin S. These fibers are surprising in that the replacement of a single amino acid on the surface of hemoglobin could cause the sudden appearance of a helical structure like no other one known in nature, the "sickle helix." The fibers are awesome because of their diabolical beauty—the harmony of a closely-packed helical network, but one with deadly consequences for its possessors. In order to understand the origins of sickled cells, and to address the possible treatment of sickle cell anemia by disrupting the fibers of hemoglobin S, a full understanding of the structure of the sickle helix is essential. Such an understanding may also provide insights into other diseases that arise from altered proteins.

Since the discovery of sickled cells, many other genetic diseases have been identified; but in contrast with sickle cell anemia, virtually all of the others arise from the loss or destabilization of something. It is relatively easy to imagine how a mutation can inactivate a protein or an enzyme—a key residue is replaced by a residue with different properties and the special characteristics of the enzyme are lost. More difficult to understand is how the change in just one amino acid residue can cause a protein to assemble into an intricate helical structure that did not exist at all before the mutation. We generally think of proteins as complex molecular machines that have been perfected over millions of years of evolution. Yet, the fibers of the sickling mutation of hemoglobin arose suddenly but with sufficiently "perfected" strength and rigidity to distort red cells into the characteristic sickle shape. Lurking, in a sense, within the structure of hemoglobin was the potential to release this new helix. Other surprises yet to occur or yet to be discovered may be waiting within the structures of other proteins. In some of these cases, diseases with serious ramifications for human populations may be involved, as for example in Alzheimer's disease, a severe medical condition that involves acute memory loss and impaired functions of the nervous system in large numbers of older people. Like sickle cell anemia, Alzheimer's disease is characterized by the appearance of fibrous structures (in this case, in the brain) known as paired helical filaments. Although the disease is not inherited in the direct way that sickle cell anemia is, the alteration of a protein normally found in the brain may be involved. Ultimately progress in treating sickle cell anemia may aid the development of treatments for this and other biochemical diseases.

One of the keys to understanding the role of hemoglobin in the drama of sickle cell anemia is its ability to transport oxygen cooperatively, by virtue of its T and R conformations. The same conformational transition responsible for cooperative oxygen binding in normal hemoglobin is a crucial factor in the sickling process for the mutant form, hemoglobin S. The interactions between hemoglobin S molecules which cause them to join together in the long, thin fibers responsible for distorting red cells into the diagnostic sickle shape occur predominately in the T state. Without the mutation which replaces glutamic acid with valine at just the right position to make these interactions in the T state possible, hemoglobin molecules will not form helical fibers, and the red cells will retain their natural rounded form—a partially collapsed sphere called a biconcave disk. Thus, the sickle helix of hemoglobin S in the T state is the agent of red cell sickling.

A helix is one of the chemical structures that forms naturally for long molecules or linear arrays of several molecules. Other helical structures include the double helix of DNA, which contains the hemoglobin genes, and the alpha helix, the single stranded helix already described which occurs in the structure of the hemoglobin alpha and beta chains. The sickle helix responsible for sickle cell anemia is structurally a great deal more complex than the double or alpha helix.

As scientists began to try to understand how a simple mutation was able to cause the appearance of a new and intricate structure, it was clear that detailed information about the molecular structure of the hemoglobin S fibers would be needed. A major effort has been made in the last decade to carry out studies defining the structure of the fibers of sickle cell hemoglobin more fully, especially those regions on the surface of the hemoglobin molecule that participate in various contacts between molecules in the fibers. If the portion of the hemoglobin molecule participating in a major contact could be modified chemically, there is a good chance that fiber formation could be blocked. Although the valine introduced by the primary sickle mutation would be an ideal place to attack the molecule with an antisickling reagent, valine is an extremely unreactive amino acid. Therefore, it is necessary to identify other portions of the hemoglobin molecule where more reactive targets can be found and where modifications might alter fiber formation.

When Linus Pauling and his colleagues recognized that sickling was due to an abnormality of hemoglobin, they proposed that the modified hemoglobin was assembling into an elongated structure of some kind that caused the characteristic distortion of cell shape. Shortly afterward, electron microscopists examined thin sections of sickled cells and reported the presence of narrow, rod-like structures aligned roughly with the long axis of the cells.[1] The details of the structures could not be discerned from the sectioned samples, however, because the embedding in plastic that was required to carry out the sectioning masks details considerably. Sharper images from electron microscopy can generally be achieved by using samples free of plastic that are stabilized and contrasted by the addition of heavy metal salts. Since the heavy metals reveal the outlines of the structure, in a manner similar to a footprint, this method is called negative staining. Unfortunately, for hemoglobin S fibers, negative stains cannot reveal great detail, since the size of the metal molecules are approximately 15% of the size of hemoglobin. A fair comparison would be to imagine a casting of a human body obtained by using a mold made out of grapefruits. A great deal of detail would be lost though the general outlines and orientation of the figure could be deduced. The situation is less favorable for hemoglobin, since its structure is more spherical than the human body. Even deductions regarding its orientation are difficult to obtain. Nevertheless, electron microscopy with negative staining seemed the best strategy when my colleagues and I began studying the structure of the fibers in the early 1970s. Eventually this approach yielded information that, when combined with our knowledge of hemoglobin structure from other sources, enabled us to achieve significant progress in describing the structure of the fibers.

The first goal was to determine the overall positioning of the hemoglobin S molecules. A number of experimental difficulties were faced. Hemoglobin is normally present in cells at extremely high concentrations, and the concentration is often augmented to even higher levels in sickle cells. However, successful studies with negative stain involve very dilute preparations. Moreover, the fibers are unstable once removed from the highly concentrated environment of the red cells. Fibers can be formed from purified hemoglobin by raising the concentration, but once fibers form, the solution gels to form a solid mass that is difficult to handle. In addition, since fiber formation only occurs readily with hemoglobin S in the T state, and since the T state predominates only in the absence of oxygen, special care must be taken to carry out all of the experiments under conditions which rigorously exclude exposure to air. Eventually various techniques were developed which permitted fibers stabilized by negative stain to be obtained directly from cells (Fig. 6.1), as well as gels, yielding richly detailed images of individual fibers (Fig. 6.2A).

Images of the fibers obtained by electron microscopy revealed an unusual complexity compared with other helical structures previously studied (principally by Aaron Klug and his colleagues, who pioneered the development of image reconstruction methods for electron microscopy). The fibers did not possess a cylindrical or tubular structure, as had been expected, but were complicated by a periodic variation in diameter in individual images, as seen in Figure 6.2A. In addition, the absence of a darkly staining core, as had been observed for tubular structures, suggested that the fibers of hemoglobin S had a solid core. Because of this complexity, the details of the fiber structure could be determined only

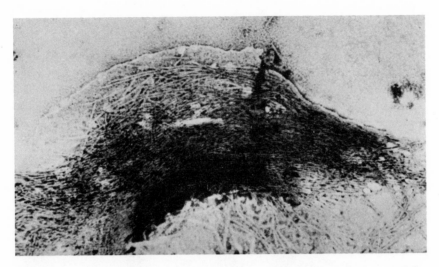

Figure 6.1. A sickled cell that has been lysed with negative stain to reveal the fibers aligned to form the tip of the cell.

with special computer methods, and developing suitable programs took considerable time.

Some five years after we began working with hemoglobin S fibers, G. Dykes, R. Crepeau, and I were able to report a full, three-dimensional structure for the fibers.[2] We discovered that each fiber was made up of 14 strands of hemoglobin S molecules bound together like beads on a string (Figs. 6.2B-D, 6.3A). The arrangement of the 14 strands explained the periodic variation in diameter. Since the fiber cross-section has an elliptical shape, with a wide diameter corresponding to five strands and a narrow diameter corresponding to four strands, the images display wide and narrow profiles caused by the twist of the helix. In addition, the location of strands in the center of the structure explained why the images did not have a hollow appearance. Overall, the strands were wound together tightly into a helical cable, with 4 strands on the inside and 10 strands on the outside (Fig. 6.2B-D).

When we tried to deduce the orientation of the hemoglobin molecules within the 14-strand structure, we discovered that no simple pattern of interactions between hemoglobin S molecules existed which could explain why the presence of the valine at the beta-6 position joined the molecules together in fibers. Since strands occurred at both inner and outer positions, there appeared to be a large variety of different classes of contacts between molecules. As a result, it was initially difficult to understand how the single beta-6 mutation could be responsible for such a complex structure. However, we had noticed the occasional occurrence of fibers with a slightly different appearance; when these minor forms were analyzed, we found the same general overall structure as the 14-strand fibers, but with the difference that certain of the strands were missing. Moreover, the strands were always missing in pairs, and always involved the same pairing. We therefore concluded that pairs of strands were a basic feature of

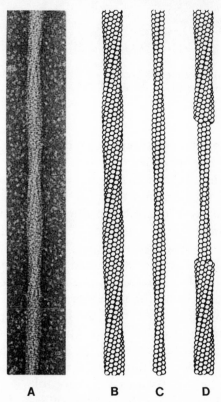

A   B   C   D

Figure 6.2. (A) Sickle cell hemoglobin fiber as imaged by an electron microscope for a negatively stained sample; the average diameter of the fibers is 200 Å (ten billion Å = 1 meter). (B) Model of the outer 10 strands with each ball representing a molecule of hemoglobin S. (C) Model of the inner 4 strands. (D) Composite model indicating the juxtaposition of the inner and outer strands.

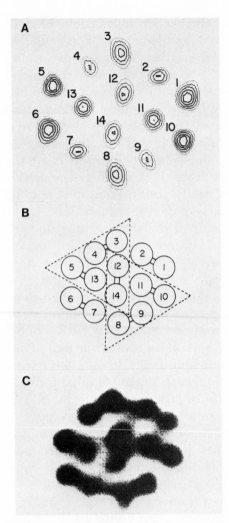

Figure 6.3. Cross sections of a sickle cell hemoglobin fiber. (A) Reconstruction of a negatively stained fiber showing the locations of the 14 strands. (B) A model for the pairing of the strands deduced from incomplete fibers. (C) Reconstruction from an embedded fiber which supports the pairing scheme presented in B in terms of the proximity of individual strands within pairs.

the structure, such that the fibers could be described as a helix composed of seven double-strands (Fig. 6.3B).[3]

Recently, we have succeeded in improving our embedding procedures, and as a result have obtained images of sections that show considerable detail. (Negatively stained fibers are generally slightly distorted by interactions with the negative stain and the supporting material, but embedded fibers have the advantage of being stabilized by the plastic matrix.) Analysis of the fibers reveals pairs of strands whose two members are significantly closer together to each other than to other strands (Fig. 6.3C). Therefore, these latest studies confirm that the basic organization of the sickle helix consists of double strands.

When we examined the spacings of hemoglobin S molecules within the double strands that make up the sickle helix, we observed that all seven pairs in each fiber were approximately half-staggered, that is, the two strands were out of register with one another by a distance equal to half the diameter of a hemoglobin molecule. If we picture the strands running vertically, the hemoglobin molecules of each strand are halfway above or below the molecules of the opposite strand of the pair. This arrangement of double strands was especially interesting, because a number of years earlier a similar arrangement of strands had been detected in a crystalline form of hemoglobin S by B. Wishner, W. Love, and their colleagues.[4] Most of our knowledge of the molecular structure of proteins has come from x-ray diffraction studies of crystals of purified proteins. Because x-rays have a wavelength comparable to the dimensions of atoms, they are especially useful for studying molecular structure.

Initially, there was no reason to expect the crystals to be related to the fibers, since the crystals were prepared under much different conditions than exist in sickled cells. However, several aspects of the structure suggested a similarity between the arrangement of hemoglobin S molecules in these crystals and in the sickle helix. First, in spectral studies with polarized light it appeared that the orientation of the hemoglobin S molecules in the double strands of the crystals was very similar to the orientation of the hemoglobin S molecules in the fibers. Moreover, within the double strands of the crystal, each molecule of hemoglobin S binds to the molecule in the opposite strand via one of its beta-6 valines (Fig. 6.4). In this way the two strands are linked, with each hemoglobin mol-

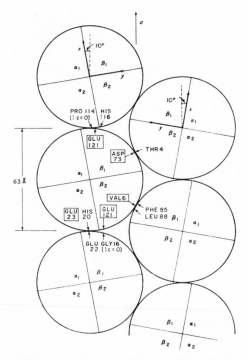

Figure 6.4. Schematic representation of the double strand of hemoglobin S found in crystals. Each molecule contributes its beta 6 valine to the contact with the molecule of the opposite strand diagonally below. In addition, each molecule has a receptor pocket involving positions beta 85 and 88 to accept the valine from the molecule of the opposite strand diagonally above. Positions beta 23 and 121 participate in the contacts along individual strands. (From Wishner, Ward, Lattman, and Love, 1975.)

ecule "donating" a valine to the molecule across and (in the orientation illustrated) below and "receiving" a valine from the molecule across and above. The receiving site is a pocket made up of nonpolar amino acids (beta-85 phenylalanine and beta-88 leucine) of the "other" beta chain, that is, the beta chain that does not contribute the beta-6 valine. In addition, for a number of contact points between molecules in the crystals, evidence indicated that similar contact points existed in the fibers, since mutant forms of hemoglobin with amino acid replacements at these sites had been studied and found to exhibit strengthened or weakened fiber stability. For these reasons, and because of a resemblance between the x-ray diffraction patterns of the crystals and patterns obtained for partially ordered arrays of the fibers by B. Magdoff-Fairchild and her collaborators, the crystals were concluded to have some essential features in common with the fibers. The presence of half-staggered double strands as the main unit in both structures gave added support to this view. Therefore, we began to formulate models for the fibers based on their similarity with the crystals. The orientation in the crystals predicted the structure and orientation of the hemoglobin S molecules in the fibers in far greater detail than could the images revealed by electron microscopy alone.[5]

The first step in the development of a model of the fibers was to clarify the exact relationship between the crystals and the fibers. While the studies on the crystals of hemoglobin S were extremely informative, it was apparent that the orientation of hemoglobin S molecules would have to be adjusted to convert the strands from their linear form in the crystals to the helical form of the fibers. The exact movements required for this conversion and the resulting placement of the hemoglobin molecules at the various positions of the fibers were deduced. Essentially only the surface of the hemoglobin S molecules in the T state plays a part in fiber formation. The important contact regions can be located on the surface of a hemoglobin molecule in much the same way that geographical locations are specified on the surface of the earth. Surface maps of hemoglobin can be calculated by converting the positions of the hemoglobin atoms into polar coordinates and defining their positions in terms of "longitude" and "latitude" (Fig. 6.5). In addition, "altitudes" were calculated to determine which atoms were too far from the surface to participate in the contacts.

In order to visualize a complete strand of the sickle helix, we can imagine the spheres stacked, with the "south pole" of one molecule on the "north pole" of the molecule below. In this respect, the strands represent a heterologous association, in the terminology of Monod discussed in the previous chapter. A similar map was constructed for the "back side" of the hemoglobin surface, which involves mainly alpha chains. On the map shown in Figure 6.5, involving mainly beta chains, the boxes with names refer to the position of hemoglobin mutants that have been tested for their influence on the formation of fibers when combined with the sickle mutation. The boxes made of solid lines (as for Korle Bu, Pyrgos, Memphis, and so on) refer to mutants that alter sick-

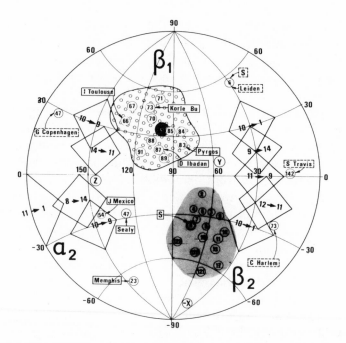

Figure 6.5. Hemoglobin structure presented as a surface map in polar coordinates. Interactions to form single strands of the fiber would occur with the "north pole" of one molecule in contact with the "south pole" of the molecule above. Positions around the S mutation (beta 6) that participate in double-strand formation are shaded in the lower portion of the structure. The positions that form the receptor site in the upper portion of the structure (around beta 85) are outlined in the motif with circles. The numbers in the diamond-shaped areas refer to the positions that contribute to the various contacts between strands, with the numbering of strands as in Figure 6.3B. Names in continuous boxes refer to known mutations of hemoglobin that interfere with fiber formation in combination with hemoglobin S. Names in dashed boxes do not alter fiber formation. (From Edelstein, 1981.)

ling, while the boxes made of dashed lines (as for G Copenhagen, S Travis, Leiden, C Harlem, and the "other" location of the S mutation) refer to mutants that do not influence sickling. The position of the Korle Bu mutation, beta-73, was one of the first locations identified where a second mutation alters the effect of the sickle mutation. We now understand that this effect arises from the location of the beta-73 position close to the receptor pocket.

Locating positions on a map of the surface permits visualization of the interactions critical to the formation of fibers in sickled cells. The first major conclusion from such an analysis concerned the role of valine. Its participation in the criss-crossing interactions between paired strands revealed for the first time why this single amino acid change leads to cell sickling. If the valine is not present to stabilize the strands by linking them together, the strands are not sufficiently stable to remain intact. Thus, for normal hemoglobin, no strands are formed in significant quantities, and the molecules remain in the free, unassociated state.

When strands form from hemoglobin S in the T state, each hemoglobin molecule contributes only one of its two beta-6 valines to a contact with another molecule—the valine below the "equator" on the surface maps contacts the receptor pocket of the molecule in the opposite strand of the double strand. The portion of the hemoglobin molecule that "receives" the critical valine from the opposite strand is above the "equator" at the site of the beta-85 receptor pocket. Thus, each molecule donates a valine to the opposite molecule slightly below (in the orientation depicted) in the double strand and receives a valine in its receptor pocket from the molecule slightly above.

A more detailed model of the hemoglobin molecule can be obtained with the use of computer graphics. In the model shown in Figure 6.6, each amino acid is represented by a sphere, with the beta chain in darker shades. The location of the receptor pocket is indicated by the beta-73 position, while the beta-6 indicates the position of the key valine residue. In the R state, the beta chains are closer together and the proper positioning for the donor and receptor pockets is disturbed. This explains why the sickle helix readily forms only for molecules of hemoglobin S in the T state.

In addition to the hydrophobic interactions between the strands of each double strand, sets of interactions exist between different double strands. The locations of these interactions on the surface of the hemoglobin S molecules are indicated by the diamond shaped areas containing numbers in Figure 6.5. The numbers refer to the positions of the strands, as indicated in the "end-on" view presented in Figure 6.3B. The number before the arrow indicates the strand on which one partner in the contact is found, and the number after the arrow indicates the strand on which the other partner in the contact is found. Interactions between the double strands for the most part involve charged amino

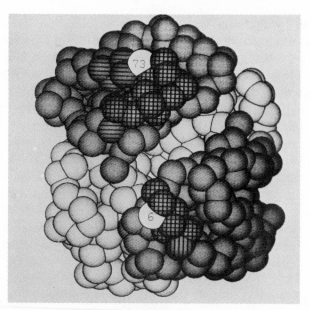

Figure 6.6. Space-filling model of hemoglobin, orientated as in Figure 6.5. Each sphere corresponds to an amino acid residue. Darker spheres are for the beta chains, lighter spheres are for the alpha chains. The positions of the beta 6 valine that participates in the contact between strands is indicated by the "6" on the lower beta chain, and the regions of the receptor site that binds the valine of the molecule diagonally above on the opposite strand are indicated by the "73" on the upper beta chain.

acids linked in salt bridges. Additional interactions have been located on the other side of the hemoglobin S molecule, involving mainly alpha chains. An overall view of the interactions between strand pairs is presented in Figure 6.7. In principle, if any of the major contacts between double strands could be interrupted by chemical modification, sickling could be prevented or diminished. Such an interruption of fiber structure has been demonstrated in laboratory studies to occur with certain "double mutants" of hemoglobin formed from beta chains carrying the sickle mutation and alpha chains carrying mutations that lie at certain contacts. For several of these double mutants, fiber formation is greatly reduced compared with hemoglobin S alone. Therefore, if a similar change could be induced chemically on the hemoglobin S molecules, the condition of individuals with sickle cell anemia could be significantly improved. Strategies along these lines are one of the possibilities that will be discussed more fully in Chapter 8.[6]

One perspective that I would like to emphasize concerns the remarkable intricacy that arises in the 14-strand structure of hemoglobin S as a consequence of the replacement of glutamic acid by valine. The reason this mutation generates a new structure may be related to the slight tendency of normal hemoglobin molecules to form single strands. The beta-6 valine lies near −30 degrees latitude on the surface map for the molecules in the orientation found in the strands. This location corresponds exactly to the required position for joining strands in the most stable arrangement—a staggering of the strands by half the diameter of the hemoglobin S molecules. In addition, the presence of a hydrophobic "receptor" pocket at +30 degrees latitude provides the

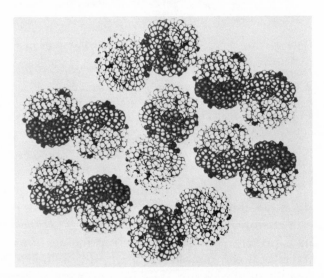

Figure 6.7. Molecular model of an end-on view of the hemoglobin S fibers. The spacing between double strands is exaggerated to illustrate strand pairing. The hemoglobin molecules are represented as in Figure 6.6, with one sphere per amino acid residue and beta chains darker than alpha chains. However, the perspective of this figure corresponds to the molecule in the preceding figure viewed from above; therefore, the beta 6 Val site is buried in the contact between pairs of molecules of each double strand. Of the seven pairs of double strands, the three that are intersected by a vertical line at the center of the figure have a polarity opposite to that of the other four. (From Rodgers, Crepeau, and Edelstein, 1986.)

other essential ingredient in holding the strands in pairs. Once this interaction is present, the pairs have sufficient stability and the complete helix with seven pairs of strands is formed.

We should also note that sickling is possible because hemoglobin is present in red cells at extremely high concentrations. So as to achieve such high solubility, the surface evolved to be highly charged. The loss of one charge due to the sickle mutation thus significantly lowers solubility and drives the hemoglobin S molecules to associate into fibers. Studies with other mutant hemoglobins and chemically modified hemoglobins are currently being carried out to determine if associations between molecules can be induced by other factors. Hemoglobins from other species might also be useful. For example, the hemoglobin of deer forms fibers that distort the cell structure under certain conditions. However, for deer hemoglobin, fibers occur only in the R state and do not appear to interfere significantly with circulation. Therefore, deer hemoglobin is not a particularly instructive model for human hemoglobin S.

From the results described here, we now have a fairly complete understanding of the sickle helix. Using special correlation techniques, we have recently obtained enhanced images from the electron microscope that display the sickle helix in its full diabolic beauty (Fig. 6.8). The strand at the front side of the sickle helix progresses up to the right (making it a "right-handed" helix), but in the electron microscope the front and back surfaces are superimposed. As a result, a series of crossing lines are seen and it is not possible in a single image to distinguish aspects of the structure from the front and the back. Molecules aligned as in the spiral network seen in the figure produce many such sickle helicies in the red blood cells of individuals homozygous for hemoglobin S, with the resulting anemia and severely impaired circulation. Nevertheless, for any particular cell, whether or not sickling occurs remains a complicated process, which includes another important factor, time. It is this factor that we must consider now in order to complete our understanding of the formation of the sickle helix and its role in cell sickling.

The difficulties in blood circulation arising from sickled cells are probably most serious in the capillary beds of various parts of the body. At such points the blood vessels are often just wide enough to permit one red cell at a time to move through, releasing

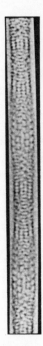

Figure 6.8. A negatively stained fiber, enhanced by correlation methods, which reveals in detail many features of the helical structure. (From Rodgers, Crepeau, and Edelstein, 1986.)

oxygen from its hemoglobin as it passes. Once its hemoglobin is predominately in a deoxygenated T state, the cell is subject to sickling if the individual is homozygous SS. The distorted sickle shape of the cell can then cause clogging in the narrow capillary. Since the transit time of cells through capillaries is a matter of seconds, we can see that cells are in a race to get through the capillaries and into the larger veins, which are less susceptible to clogging, before sickling starts. If cells begin to sickle while still in the capillaries, their transit will be slowed down, more oxygen will be removed, more molecules will assume the T conformation, and more sickling will be provoked. Other cells entering the capillary may also be slowed, leading to their sickling as well.

The time it takes for a cell to sickle is thus a critical factor in the problems associated with sickling. Sickling time for individual cells, studied by Colleta, Ferrone, Hofrichter, and Eaton using elegant laser methods, was found to occur mainly in the time range from 0.01 to 1.0 second. The higher the concentration of hemoglobin S in the cells, the more easily (and more rapidly) fiber formation can be initiated and the shorter the delay in sickling. Cells that take longest to sickle would have a good chance of getting through a capillary before sickling occurs. However, if they get stuck behind a cell with a higher concentration of hemoglobin S and a shorter delay, there may be time for even the cells with long delays to begin sickling.[7]

The reasons that a single change in the hemoglobin beta chains can lead to such a range of sickling times arise from certain special properties of sickled cells. First of all, the population of red cells in an individual with sickle cell anemia is much more varied than that found in a normal individual. In general, red cells range from "young" to "old," with the vast majority in between these extremes. Older cells contain more hemoglobin per unit of volume and are therefore more dense. Younger cells, called reticulocytes, are still in the process of making hemoglobin and therefore contain less hemoglobin per unit volume than mature red cells. For sickle cells, this distribution by age is more pronounced. The anemia associated with sickling pushes red cell production to its limits and leads to a larger population of younger cells. At the other extreme, there are many more very dense cells than in normal blood, apparently because repeated sickling damages the cell membrane, permitting a leakage of ions and water and causing a progressive dehydration that concentrates the hemoglobin S molecules. Although the sickled cell is often referred to as though it were a well-defined entity, the population of sickled cells is actually a very heterogeneous mixture of cells with different concentrations of hemoglobin. The range of hemoglobin concentration in sickled cells can be measured by separating the cells using centrifugation on density gradients; the cells with the highest concentrations of hemoglobin descend to near the bottom of the gradients where the density is highest, while the cells with lower concentrations distribute at higher positions where the density is lower.[8]

Studies with solutions of purified hemoglobin S have revealed that the time for fiber formation (and hence sickling) is extremely sensitive to the concentration of hemoglobin. An increase of just 1% in the concentration of hemoglobin in a cell may result in a decrease of 30% in the time required for fiber formation. Such effects help to explain why individuals with sickle cell trait rarely experience cell sickling. The lower concentration of hemoglobin S in the cells of these AS heterozygous individuals leads to sickling times that are thousands of times slower than those for SS cells—too slow for sickling to occur to a significant extent during passage through capillaries.

Detailed studies of the rate of fiber formation for a wide range of conditions have revealed that the mechanism of fiber formation and growth involves two distinct processes. First, individual hemoglobin molecules must associate in order to initiate formation of the first fibers. This process presumably begins with the assembly of a very short "seed" or "nucleus" of the 14-strand sickle helix. Association of individual molecules of hemoglobin S to form such nuclei is called "homogeneous nucleation." The nuclei are difficult to form, but once present, hemoglobin S molecules can readily add on to form a complete fiber. Once one fiber has formed, additional fibers can form more easily by using the existing fiber as a template. This second type of process in which one fiber helps to initiate the formation of another is called "heterogeneous nucleation." The two types of nucleation are illustrated in Figure 6.9.[9]

In the illustration of heterogeneous nucleation, the new fiber is shown growing parallel to the original fiber. In sickled cells, fibers

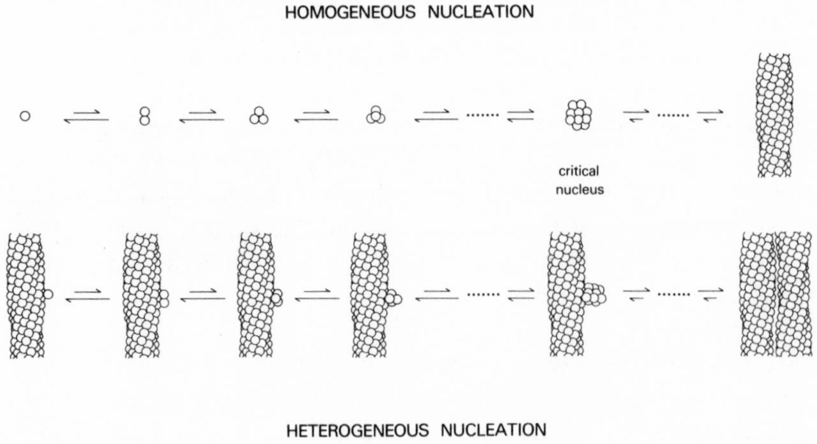

Figure 6.9. Homogeneous and heterogeneous nucleation mechanisms for formation of hemoglobin S fibers. (From Ferrone, Hofrichter, and Eaton, 1985.)

in close parallel packing of this type are often encountered, aligned with the regions of wide and narrow diameters of each fiber staggered to provide complementary surfaces. In addition, elaborate fan-shaped or "holly-leaf" patterns are also encountered in sickled cells, arising from layers of single fibers that are superimposed, with each layer rotated by 26 degrees relative to the next layer (Fig. 6.10). This rotation corresponds precisely to the packing expected for alignment by interpenetration of the helical grooves of fibers of adjacent layers (Fig. 6.11). Alignment of fibers with the 26-degree angle may be responsible for the fact that cells of hemoglobin S are indeed sickle shaped, with the ends sometime showing highly pronounced curvature (Fig. 6.12). Therefore, when heterogeneous nucleation occurs, it may involve the 26-degree orientation, as well as the parallel orientation.[10]

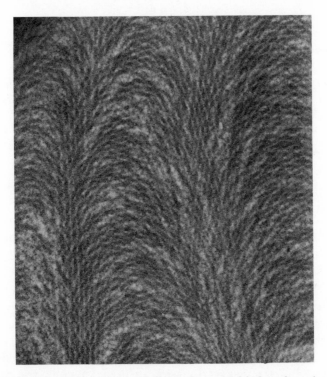

Figure 6.10. Fan-shaped sheets of fibers. In embedded and sectioned cells, each superimposed layer of fibers is rotated by 26 degrees with respect to the line of fiber alignment in the adjacent layer.

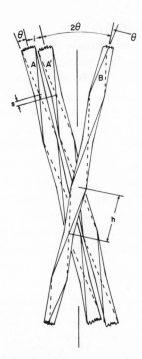

Figure 6.11. Fiber interdigitation. The angle of 26 degrees arises from the fact that the helical grooves of each fiber lie at an angle (theta) of 13 degrees with respect to the fiber axis. The interpenetration of the "back" face of the fibers of one layer with the "front" of the next layer of fibers leads to a relative orientation of twice theta, or 26 degrees. (From Edelstein and Crepeau, 1979.)

The relative importance of the two types of nucleation, homogeneous and heterogeneous, depends on the concentration of hemoglobin. The higher the concentration, the easier for homogeneous nucleation to be achieved. When the concentration of hemoglobin is relatively low, a long time (many seconds) will be required for the formation of the first fiber, but once formed, many other fibers will be initiated by the heterogeneous mechanism. In contrast, for higher concentrations, many fibers can be formed quickly by the homogeneous mechanism. Therefore, the higher the concentration of hemoglobin in a cell, the greater the fraction of fibers that will be formed by homogeneous nucleation. For the highest concentrations found in sickle cells, the majority of fibers will be formed by homogeneous nucleation.

The problems caused by sickling cells are increased by the fact that not all cells unsickle upon oxygenation. For the most dense cells, fibers persist even while the red cells are in the lungs, where oxygen concentrations are the highest. There are several factors responsible for this. First, fiber formation by hemoglobin S stabilizes the T state, so that oxygen affinity is lower for sickle cells than for normal cells. Therefore, even at the oxygen concentration of the lungs, the full allosteric transition may not be completed and a portion of the molecules will remain in the T state, which naturally forms fibers. Second, the high hemoglobin S concentrations found in the most dense cells gives added stability to the fibers and hence results in extremely low oxygen affinity. And finally, in individuals with sickle cell anemia, progressive damage to the lungs reduces the volume of oxygen available, so that oxygen concentrations in the arterial blood are below normal values. As a result of these factors, a certain fraction of the red cells in individuals with sickle cell anemia are irreversibly sickled. Noguchi and Schechter have used nuclear magnetic resonance techniques to demonstrate directly that an appreciable fraction of fibers remain in certain sickled cells even when they are almost fully oxygenated.[11]

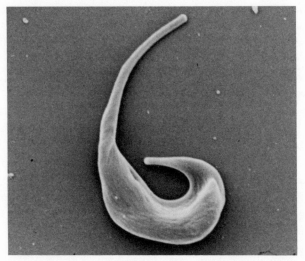

Figure 6.12. A highly curved sickle cell. The fact that sickled cells are rarely rod-like emphasizes the importance of oblique interactions between fibers of the type described in the previous figure. (From Franck et al., 1985. Reproduced from the *Journal of Clinical Investigation* by copyright permission of the American Society for Clinical Investigation.)

From this discussion of fiber formation and its consequences in sickling cells, we can appreciate how the simple mutation that changes one hemoglobin residue can lead to a variety of cellular manifestations. This variation at the cellular level helps to explain why the clinical symptoms of sickle cell anemia discussed in Chapter 3 cover such a wide range. Additional factors which can moderate severity are discussed in the following chapter.

We can also now summarize more fully what constellation of factors led to the proliferation of the S gene in Africa, first in malaria-resistant AS carriers and then in increasing numbers of homozygous SS individuals. Although the red cells of AS heterozygotes do not usually sickle (since the normal hemoglobin interferes with the formation of fibers by hemoglobin S), the AS cells can sickle if unusually low levels of oxygen occur in the red cells. Then, the T state will predominate for both hemoglobins, and some fiber formation with sickling will occur. Studies indicate that malaria parasites in the red cells of AS individuals trigger some sickling by excreting acidic waste products. Acidification would drive the hemoglobin molecules into the T state, permitting the fibers responsible for sickling to form. Such sickled cells ultimately inhibit the development of the invading organism, though the exact mechanism is not known. Because sickled cells are more fragile than normal cells, they may simply be destroyed in the spleen before the parasites complete the stage in their life cycle that takes place in the red cells. As a result, the malaria does not progress. Alternatively, the sickling—which is known to make the red cells leaky—may result in the loss of some ion such as potassium that the parasites require for growth, and this too would prevent the progression of the infection. In either case, the fact that predominantly T state (deoxygenated) molecules form fibers in sickle cell disease is an essential aspect. Had it been the R state, formation of fibers would not be promoted by parasite growth in the red cells, and natural selection of the sickle trait would not have occurred.[12]

While elucidation of the exact mechanism whereby parasite growth is inhibited in AS cells will require additional studies, the basic principles now seem clear. Individuals carrying a sickle mutation had slightly better chances than individuals with normal hemoglobin for survival in environments where malaria was a threat. Over time, the percentage of individuals with sickle trait could reach the levels found in malaria-infested regions of Africa—25% for the Igbos, with similar values found across the central tropics into Zaire, where an incidence of 30% has been reported for the baLuba. At this incidence, more than 2% of all the children born to the baLuba will be homozygous for hemoglobin S and suffer from sickle cell anemia.

Because the source of this disease is at the level of DNA, it is to this level that scientists are beginning to turn to develop new strategies for diagnosis and treatment of the growing numbers of afflicted.

CONFRONTING SICKLING AT THE GENES

$\mathbf{T}$he threats to human existence from natural causes have become physically smaller and smaller since the first appearance of human beings on earth. Our early ancestors were in danger of death principally from animal predators. As population densities increased, viruses, microbes, and parasites replaced predators as our most serious enemies. Today, more human beings are afflicted with malaria than with any other illness. Modern drugs and antibiotics, as well as immunizations, have lessened the threat of infectious diseases in many parts of the world; but illnesses caused by invading organisms, especially parasites, remain major health hazards in Africa. In recent years, we have begun to recognize and define the risks of exposure to entities in the environment even smaller than viruses—single molecules which can trigger the cancerous mutations that appear with disturbing frequency in the DNA of our own genetic systems. Finally, we are beginning to face the spontaneous mutations that are an intrinsic feature of our genetic systems—mutations that can ultimately lead to diseases such as sickle cell anemia.

Because sickle cell anemia is caused by a permanent change in one base of the beta-globin gene, the only way to "cure" sickle cell anemia would be to eliminate it at the source—in the DNA. Intervention of this type is a dream held out for genetic engineering, but as yet the means of realizing this dream are not apparent. A harmless virus might be engineered to deliver a corrected gene, but we know of no way to ensure that it would be inserted reliably in the chromosome to replace the sickle mutation. In addition, a bone marrow transplant would accomplish the same objective, by replacing cells producing hemoglobin S with cells producing normal hemoglobin, but it is extremely unlikely that this approach will be adopted on a large scale in the foreseeable future. The obstacles are overwhelming, including the difficulty of finding a suitable donor for each patient, the high risk to the patient during the period when the immunological system must be suppressed, and the enormous expenditures of resources and manpower needed for each transplant.[1] Rather than trying to cure the disease by eliminating the cause, current efforts are directed toward relieving the symptoms, principally by modifying hemoglobin S (see Chapter 8). However, an attack at the level of DNA has recently been suggested on the basis of trials using drugs that modify the switching on of genes to produce protein. These results, as well as other aspects of sickling involving DNA, will be presented here.

Of the thousands of genes within the human cell that specify proteins, some are dormant at certain stages in the development and maturation of the body. One example is the gene for the gamma chains of fetal hemoglobin, or hemoglobin F. Like the adult form (hemoglobin A), fetal hemoglobin is composed of four subunits, including two alpha chains. However, in place of the two beta chains found in hemoglobin A, there are two gamma chains in hemoglobin F. The gene for gamma chains lies near the gene for beta chains on the human chromosome designated number 11; the gene for alpha chains resides on chromosome 16. See Figure 7.1. The presence of the gamma chains leads to a slightly stronger binding of oxygen by fetal blood than occurs with adult blood, because hemoglobin F binds poorly the cofactor 2,3 DPG which helps to lower the affinity of hemoglobin A by stabilizing the T state. As a result, fetal blood supply is assured of competing favorably with the maternal blood supply for oxygen.

Near the time of birth, synthesis of gamma globin is almost completely switched off, while synthesis of beta globin is switched on. How such switching occurs remains one of the major unsolved problems of human molecular biology. However, it has been observed that the DNA of the inactive gene tends to be more heavily methylated than the DNA of the active gene. Methylation refers to the addition of a methyl group to the ring structure of one of DNA's four classes of bases. The methylation in this case occurs on the base known as cytidine that is derived from cytosine, to form methylcytidine.

A synthetic base known as 5-azacytidine cannot be methylated at the position corresponding to the site of methylation of cytosine. Moreover, when incorporated into DNA, this compound depresses methylation levels and thereby activates some previously inactive genes. It has recently been observed that treatment of sickle cell anemia patients with 5-azacytidine (a drug commonly used to treat leukemia) causes the gamma gene to be turned on and more hemoglobin F to be produced. Adults can function well with hemoglobin F. In fact, routine screening has revealed a genetic abnormality known as "hereditary persistence of fetal hemoglobin" (or simply HPFH); studies of people with this condition

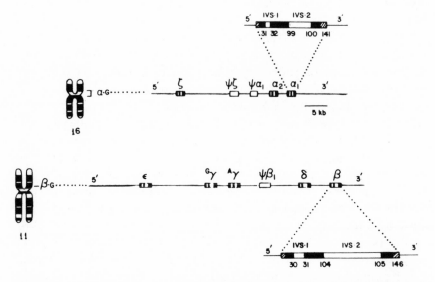

Figure 7.1. Chromosome maps for the globin genes. The alpha-globin gene family lies on chromosome 16, while the beta-globin gene family lies on chromosome 11. Expanded regions of the alpha and beta genes indicate the locations of intervening sequences (IVS). The gamma-globin genes, associated with the production of fetal hemoglobin, lie to the left of the beta-globin genes. (From Antonarakis, Kazazian, and Orkin, 1985.)

reveal that it causes no major adverse effects. Therefore, an increase in hemoglobin F production would greatly benefit sickle cell anemia patients, since hemoglobin F interferes with fiber formation by hemoglobin S and diminishes the extent of sickling.

While the idea of treating sickle cell anemia with a drug that alters DNA methylation seems to make sense, some recent experiments indicate that the original explanation for the action of 5-azacytidine may have been oversimplified. Two other cancer drugs, hydroxyurea and cytosine arabinoside, fail to alter methylation but nevertheless appear to increase levels of hemoglobin F. Red blood cells pass through many precursor stages before they mature, and these anticancer drugs (which are thought to stop the growth of dividing cells) may alter the maturation process in a way that leads to the elevated levels of fetal hemoglobin. In any case, it is too early to tell whether such drugs that act on DNA will be useful in treating sickle cell anemia. Even if they are successful for short periods, long-term application may be limited, since the drugs themselves may be carcinogenic.[2]

On the other hand, biochemical methods which can detect the presence of the mutation in the DNA that is responsible for sickling have already established their usefulness in the diagnosis of sickle cell anemia. The methods are based on the existence of enzymes found in many different species of bacteria whose function is to recognize and inactivate "foreign" DNA molecules, that is, DNA from other sources, particularly viruses, which has made its way into the cell. Each enzyme recognizes a sequence of four to seven bases in the foreign DNA and cuts the DNA at that position. The corresponding sequence in the DNA of the host bacterium escapes being cut because it is "camouflaged" by methylation. More than 100 different restriction enzymes (or restriction endonucleases, as they are also called), each recognizing and cutting a different sequence of bases, have been isolated from bacterial sources. Because many of these sequences also occur in human DNA, the restriction enzymes have provided a valuable tool in generating specific DNA "fragments" from human cells.

The sites that restriction enzymes recognize and cut in human DNA are relatively rare; consequently, when human DNA is mixed with a particular restriction enzyme, the result is a set of fragments, each beginning and ending with the particular sequence of bases that characterize the recognition site of that restriction enzyme. The various methods available to analyze such fragments have permitted individual genes to be isolated. It is this ability to isolate individual genes in the laboratory that has led to the biotechnology revolution of the last decade. Genes from higher organisms have been cloned in bacteria and the sequence of bases in individual genes determined. In some instances it has even been possible to transfer the genes back from bacteria to the cells of higher organisms, although not yet to humans. The rapid and convenient methods for determining the sequence of bases in the DNA of a gene (developed by Walter Gilbert and by Frederick Sanger and their respective colleagues) have given an enormous impetus to our understanding of gene structure and our ability to manipulate it.[3] These developments have led to a new biotechnology industry, whose successes have included the cloning of the human insulin gene and the production of human insulin in bacteria. As a result, diabetics no longer have to rely on insulins prepared from animal sources that are not identical to the human form.

A very surprising discovery was made when restriction enzymes were used in an attempt to isolate hemoglobin genes, to clone them in bacteria, and to determine the base sequence of the DNA. As was discovered in the same period for a number of other genes, the genes for both the alpha and beta chains of hemoglobin are not continuous, as previously assumed, but are each interrupted at two positions by stretches of DNA that do not code for amino acids in the sequences of the hemoglobin chains. These introns (or intervening sequences, briefly discussed in Chapter 5), were initially discovered in the hemoglobin genes of the rabbit and the mouse, but were soon found to occur in humans and all other vertebrate species examined. The first intervening sequence (abbreviated IVS-1) occurs in the DNA after the bases coding for the 30th amino acid in the beta chain; it is 130 bases long in humans. In the same gene, IVS-2 occurs after the bases coding for the 104th amino acid and in humans is 850 bases long. In all vertebrate species studied, IVS-2 in the beta chain gene is a much longer sequence than IVS-1, though the exact numbers of bases vary from species to species. For alpha chains, the intervening sequences occur after bases coding for the 31st and 99th amino acid positions; in humans, each is about 130 bases in length.[4] Since a splicing of messenger RNA molecules is carried out by cells to eliminate the introns, continuous polypeptides are produced with no trace of the fact that their corresponding genes were interrupted.

Introns have now been discovered in a great many genes of higher organisms, but it has not always been clear what function they play, though it is clear that they do not code for proteins. In the case of antibody molecules, it has become apparent that the regions specified by different exons (the part of the gene that is expressed) can be combined in various ways to lead to the production of many different kinds of antibodies with varied specific binding sites. Through this mechanism the immune system is capable of recognizing an extremely large number of different antigens. Hence, the presence of distinct exons appears to be an indispensable feature of the antibody-producing system. For hemoglobin, it has been suggested that different exons correspond to different functional domains of the hemoglobin molecule; for example, the central exon of the globin genes might provide the portions of the polypeptide chain that bind the heme group. Evidence in support of this hypothesis has been obtained by isolating the protein fragment coded for by the central exon region and finding that it could bind heme. It would thus seem plausible that in early evolution the distinct regions that now comprise the three exons were brought together to form a precursor gene for hemoglobin. However, for a number of other genes broken into exons, no such functional distinctions in terms of domains for their corresponding proteins are apparent and more information will be needed before the full significance of introns can be comprehended.[5]

One of the more recently characterized restriction nucleases, *Mst*II, cuts DNA wherever the sequence CCTNAGG appears (where N can be any of the four bases: A, T, G, or C). A site of attack for *Mst*II is a sequence of seven bases (CCTGAGG) in the DNA of the normal beta-globin gene. However, the sickle mutation transforms this sequence to CCTGTGG, causing the chromosome to lose one of the sites that can be cut with the *Mst*II restriction enzyme. This fact can be exploited to detect the presence of the sickle mutation.

In tests for the sickle mutation, a sample of DNA is cut with *Mst*II wherever a CCTNAGG occurs. The resulting fragments are migrated in an electric field on a porous material that separates them according to size. The fragments are then transferred to a thin filter to which a DNA probe is added for the purpose of detecting only the fragments that carry the beta-globin gene. This probe is a radioactively-labeled DNA fragment containing the beginning of the beta-globin gene; it is produced in *E. coli* through cloning. When the sample is placed in alkaline conditions to cause the two strands of the DNA double helix to separate, the probe binds some of the unlabeled sequences. Following incorporation of the probe, an x-ray film is placed on the filter. After exposing for several days, the film is developed and bands appear at the position occupied by the beta-globin gene; these bands are caused by disintegration of the radioactive probe. By comparing the positions of "standards" of DNA of known length with the position of the fragment containing the beta-globin gene, the size of the restriction fragment carrying the beta-globin gene can be estimated, as described below.

When this gene analysis is carried out, the beginning of the normal beta-globin gene is found on a *Mst*II restriction fragment containing approximately 1,200 bases, or 1.2 kilobases (abbreviated kb). DNA harboring the sickle mutation, on the other hand, produces a larger restriction fragment, a 1.4-kb fragment, because one *Mst*II site is lost as a result of the mutation. The difference in locations of the 1.2-kb and the 1.4-kb fragments are readily determined, as demonstrated by Kan and by Orkin and their respective coworkers.[6] Therefore, with this test, the presence or absence of the sickle mutation can be readily verified (Fig. 7.2).

The major advantage of a test for sickle cell anemia using DNA is that it can be applied to fetal cells obtained by amniocentesis (a procedure which involves passing a thin needle through the abdominal wall of the pregnant woman and removing a sample of amniotic fluid from the sac surrounding the fetus). When the fetus's mother and father are both carriers of the sickle mutation, examination of the *Mst*II restriction fragments from the DNA of the fetal cells can be used to determine which of the three possible hemoglobin combinations the fetus has inherited: AA (only the 1.2-kb fragment), AS (both the 1.2-kb and 1.4-kb fragments), or SS (only the 1.4-kb fragment). In the case of SS, the parents may wish to consider terminating the pregnancy.

Amniocentesis is not performed until the sixteenth week of the pregnancy because prior to that time not enough amniotic fluid exists to make the test safe and reliable. However, a new method

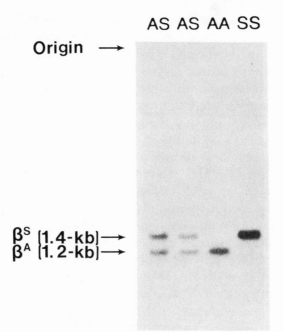

Figure 7.2. Restriction enzyme analysis of DNA for prenatal diagnosis. The presence of the 1.2-kb fragment indicates an AA individual, the 1.4-kb fragment indicates an SS individual, and both 1.2-kb and 1.4-kb fragments indicate an AS individual. (Adapted from Chang and Kan, 1982. Reprinted by permission of the *New England Journal of Medicine.*)

of prenatal diagnosis which can be performed between eight and ten weeks of pregnancy is being tested. In this case, a thin catheter or biopsy forceps is passed through the cervix and cells from the chorionic villi (small hairlike projections of the membrane that surrounds the embryo until the tenth week of pregnancy) are obtained. DNA from these cells is used in the restriction enzyme analysis of the beta-globin gene. The advantage of this test is that abortion is safer and less traumatic at an earlier stage of pregnancy, should a woman choose this option. Initial results with chorionic biopsy had indicated that the procedure had more risks of miscarriage than amniocentesis, but as more data have accumulated, the results have substantially improved.[7]

Diagnosis of sickle cell anemia in fetuses could, in principle, be used to reduce greatly the incidence of individuals born with sickle cell anemia in the future. However, this strategy has a number of drawbacks that are likely to limit its usefulness. For a variety of personal reasons, mothers and fathers may oppose abortion, and various political, social, and economic factors may complicate its implementation. Second, both parents must be aware of their status as carriers, and this knowledge may not be available or acted upon early enough to carry out amniocentesis. Third, when a fetus is positively diagnosed as SS, the physicians and health specialists counseling the parents may have difficulty in formulating, even in their own minds, the degree of difficulty that sickle cell anemia is likely to impose on the prospective child. In spite of the fact that sickle cell anemia arises from a simple genetic mutation, the clinical symptoms vary greatly, with some individuals experiencing relatively benign manifestations of the disease. There has been a vigorous effort to identify other factors that may be responsible for this variability. Recent investigations suggest that the number of alpha genes present in the chromosomes of individuals with sickle cell anemia may be one such factor, and we shall review the evidence for the role of alpha genes later in this chapter.

Prenatal diagnosis and selective abortion are, therefore, not likely to be the solution for all parents who risk bearing children with sickle cell anemia, although they can be useful tools for family planning, particularly in the developed countries. A major role for prenatal diagnosis and selective abortion in Africa is highly unlikely, at least for the foreseeable future. Although tests need to be carried out only when both parents are carriers of sickle trait, the potential number of tests for such pregnancies in Africa would overwhelm existing resources. Furthermore, most Africans do not know if they are carriers, and abortion is not generally viewed favorably by Africans.

Reservations concerning the use of prenatal diagnosis in Africa were expressed by the Ghanian expert in sickle cell anemia, Dr. Konotey-Ahulu, in response to suggestions that the technique could be a major advance for Africa and other regions of the Third World:

> To suggest, even remotely, that amniocentesis and selective abortion is the answer to sickle cell disease in the Third World not only betrays an extraordinary naivety but also raises . . . "complex ethical issues" . . . It is one thing isolated couples, out of thousands at risk, asking for the technique (that is a matter for them), but it is

quite another matter for scientists to present the technique as the breakthrough we all are waiting for to solve the sickle cell problem in the Third World. For at-risk couples in West Africa alone 140, 000 amniocenteses per million conceptions would be required to detect all these cases of hemoglobinopathy [diseases due to altered hemoglobin molecules]. Ethics apart—and this is where the naivety comes in—with a population increase of a million every 4 months in that region alone is it not time we stopped mentioning in the same breath "this major advance" and its "public health significance"?[8]

Konotey-Ahula, in the same article, cites a number of cases of homozygous SS individuals of his acquaintance who are leading active and productive lives. These cases serve to illustrate his point that even if prenatal diagnosis on a large scale in Africa were feasible, the elimination of SS fetuses by abortion may be an overreaction in view of the successful adaptation of some SS individuals.

The potential of prenatal diagnosis and selective abortion to reduce the population with a genetic disease can be illustrated by another hemoglobin mutation, beta-thalassemia. This genetic disease, which is prevalent around the Mediterranean Sea, resembles sickle cell anemia in that carriers have some resistance to malaria. But in other respects it differs dramatically; rather than involving a modification of the beta chains as in sickle cell anemia, the production of the beta chains is greatly reduced or eliminated in beta-thalassemia. Overall, individuals who are homozygous for beta-thalassemia are much more certain of facing severe and life-threatening difficulties than individuals homozygous for hemoglobin S. As a result, in regions of Italy, Greece, and the neighboring islands where the incidence of beta-thalassemia is high, prenatal diagnosis and abortion have become routine, and the number of births of thalassemic babies has been greatly reduced. According to a summary of data compiled prior to 1981,

In Greece, where 200 new thalassemics used to be born each year, the demand for prenatal testing is increasing rapidly. In Sardinia, the birth rate of affected infants has declined from 1 in 213 in 1976 to 1 in 587 in 1979. In Ferrara [Italy], the incidence of thalassemics was 1.56 per 1000 newborns in 1970 and essentially zero in 1979. And in Cyprus, there were 18 births of thalassemic babies in 1979 instead of the expected 77 . . . figures for 1980 onwards would show an even greater impact of genetic programs than indicated here.[9]

Similar results are possible for sickle cell anemia, at least in developed countries, if parents at risk are convinced that having a child with sickle cell anemia is an unacceptable burden. However, because the severity of sickle cell anemia is not so great as to make the decision to terminate a pregnancy a foregone conclusion, and because the hope of some practical treatment in the not-too-distant future is a realistic possibility, prenatal diagnosis and abortion have not had a major effect on the number of newborns with sickle cell anemia, even in the United States. Recourse to these steps is more common in families that have already had one child with sickle cell anemia. An overall screening program is hampered by the high incidence of unwed mothers among the pregnant women at risk for an infant with the disease. As a consequence, the more significant focus for the future of sickling is on measures that can be taken to treat the symptoms of the disease once the child is born. However, before taking up such measures in the following chapter, other new insights arising from the use of restriction enzymes should be reviewed.

Before *Mst*II restriction enzymes were used to diagnose sickle cell anemia, methods based on other restriction enzymes were investigated, principally in the laboratory of Y. W. Kan. Some early success was achieved with the restriction enzyme *Hpa*I. This enzyme did not cut the DNA within the beta-globin gene, but rather produced large restriction fragments within which the beta-globin gene was incorporated. In most cases, the beta-globin gene was contained on a 7.0 or 7.6-kb fragment. However, in many of the individuals examined who were known to possess the sickle mutation, the beta-globin gene was found on a 13-kb fragment. Thus, the presence of a 13-kb *Hpa*I fragment was a marker for the sickle mutation. Unfortunately, this test could not detect all cases of sickle mutation because in some individuals the abnormal gene occurred on a 7.6-kb fragment. Because it could not be distinguished from the normal gene, prenatal diagnosis in these instances was not possible. The problem for prenatal diagnosis was solved when the *Mst*II restriction enzyme began to be used, but the appearance of the sickle mutation in beta-globin genes on both 7.6-kb and 13-kb restriction fragments has intriguing implications for the origin of sickling.

The fact that the sickle mutation was found in some individuals on a larger restriction fragment meant that there had been two mutations of their chromosome number 11. One was the "sickle" mutation at the position of the 6th amino acid of the beta chains. The other occurred in the region flanking the beta-globin gene and altered one base in the *Hpa*I recognition site, GTTAAC, that was responsible for producing the 7.6-kb fragment. Since the site was no longer attacked by the *Hpa*I restriction enzyme, the larger 13-kb fragment was produced. However, because other individuals were found possessing the sickle mutation but not the flanking mutation, these results could be interpreted as an indication that the sickle mutation arose independently on more than one occasion.

The evidence for multiple origins of the sickle mutation began in 1980 with a report by Kan and Dozy on studies of the occurrence of the 7.6-kb and 13-kb fragments from various populations of the world.[10] For Africa, the highest concentrations of the sickle cell gene occur in two distinct areas, one centered roughly about the mouth of the Niger River and the other centered roughly around the mouth of the Zaire River (formerly the Congo). In the Niger region and the surrounding areas of West Africa, the sickle mutation is carried on the 13-kb fragment. In contrast, the population nearer the Zaire River possesses exclusively the 7.6-kb fragment. The possibility that the sickle cell mutation arose independently in these two population groups appeared likely, especially when another mutation of the beta-globin gene, next to the site of the sickle mutation, was found that produces hemoglobin C. This abnormal hemoglobin occurs at levels approaching hemoglobin S for tropical African populations west of the Niger River.[11] It is likely that hemoglobin C also provides some resistance to malaria.

In the hemoglobin C mutation, the GAG codon that specifies glutamic acid at the 6th position of the beta-globin gene is replaced by the AAG codon that specifies lysine. The G-to-A mutation occurs in the base next to the one changed from A to T in the sickle mutation (replacement of the GAG codon by GTG). Hence, hemoglobin C and hemoglobin S are thought to have both arisen independently from hemoglobin A by single-base mutations. (If hemoglobin C arose from hemoglobin S, or vice versa, two-base mutations would be required, which are much less probable.) However, the hemoglobin C gene is also found on the 13-kb fragment produced by *Hpa*I restriction enzymes. Therefore, the mutation responsible for the 13-kb fragment probably arose before the mutations of hemoglobins S and C. Thus, the sickle mutation must have occurred once in an ancestor of the peoples inhabiting the Niger River basin already missing the *Hpa*I site and another time in an ancester of the Zaire peoples in the vicinity of the Zaire River possessing the *Hpa*I site. Since West Africa supplied most of the slaves that arrived in North America (while the slaves taken from the southwest African coast were more likely to go to South America), it is not surprising that for a high proportion of blacks in the United States with the sickle mutation of the beta gene, the mutation occurs on the 13-kb fragment.

Outside tropical Africa, the sickle mutation is also found in low levels among a number of populations in regions where malaria is or was endemic. In North Africa and the islands and coastal regions of southernmost Europe, the sickle mutation is found on a 13-kb fragment, suggesting that the gene diffused from West Africa via trade routes through the Sahara, which have existed since antiquity. In East Africa, the Arabian peninsula, and southern India the sickle mutation is found on the 7.6-kb fragment (Fig. 7.3). For populations with the 7.6-kb fragment, it is not possible to determine from restriction fragments whether the sickle mutation arose independently two or more times in Africa, the Middle East, or India, or diffused after a single original mutational event.

Studies completed more recently point to yet a third independent origin of the sickle mutation in Africa. By examining the patterns of fragments produced with eight different restriction enzymes, Josée Pagnier and her co-investigators confirmed the original distinction between Niger and Zaire populations (since they differed by several restriction enzyme sites) and discovered a third group from Senegal, at the western edge of Africa. Because the patterns found from Benin and Algeria are the same, it would appear that the gene migrated along a north–south axis via the well-documented trans-Saharan caravan routes. These differences provide an additional tool to aid anthropologists in establishing the places of origin of blacks dispersed throughout the Americas by slave trade and to trace the migrations of the Bantu expansion more accurately. The Senegal pattern of sickle cell anemia may be less severe because individuals with this mutation produce higher levels of hemoglobin F.[12]

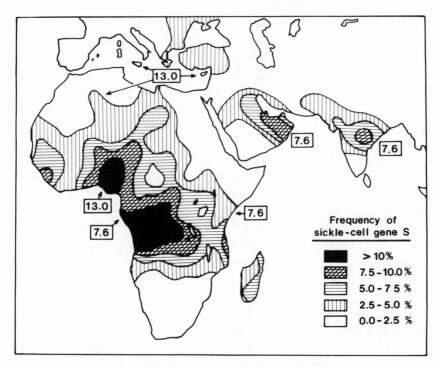

Figure 7.3. Map of original division of hemoglobin S populations into two groups based on 7.6-kb and 13-kb fragments. The unlabeled high S frequency region of Western Africa which is centered about Sierra Leone may be the origin of the "Senegalese" phenotype discovered by Pagnier and her colleagues. (Adapted from Kan and Dozy, 1980. Copyright 1980 by the AAAS.)

One additional condition of the red cell that concerns sickling directly is alpha-thalassmia. The genes for the alpha chains of hemoglobin lie on chromosome number 16 (Fig. 7.1) and have the unusual feature that two copies of the gene some 3.7-kb apart are normally present on each of these chromosomes. The typical individual therefore has four alpha genes, two on the chromosome 16 inherited from the father and an additional two on the chromosome 16 inherited from the mother. However, the absence of one or more of the alpha genes is relatively common, particularly among individuals of African descent. This condition is known as alpha-thalassemia.

Two different patterns of this disease have been recognized, principally on the basis of analyses using restriction enzyme techniques. For a particular chromosome, both copies of the alpha gene may be absent (the condition defined as alpha-thalassemia-1) or the gene may be present in only one copy (the condition defined as alpha-thalassemia-2). Alpha-thalassemia-1, if present on only one chromosome, can be tolerated, but if the alpha-thalassemia-1 condition is inherited from both parents, no alpha chains are produced and miscarriage of the fetus results. The alpha-thalassemia-1 state is limited almost exclusively to certain populations from Southeast Asia. In contrast, the alpha-thalasse-mia-2 pattern is found at a high incidence among Africans and their descendents. It occurs in nearly one of three members of the American black population. Therefore, we can assume that levels this high reflect some selective advantage conferred by the condition. As discussed in Chapter 3, beta-thalassemia is known to protect against malaria, and the same is most likely to be the case for alpha-thalassemia, given the incidence patterns we have seen. In addition, some recent studies suggest that homozygous SS patients have fewer and less severe symptoms of sickle cell anemia if they also have an alpha-thalassemia-2 gene. Conceivably, the presence of alpha-thalassemia could improve significantly the outlook for individuals with sickle cell anemia, but the outlook is clouded by a failure to find improvement in all studies.[13]

If the hypothesis that alpha-thalassemia in conjunction with sickle cell anemia leads to a reduction of the problems associated with sickling, a greater survival rate would be expected for homozygous SS individuals with alpha-thalassemia compared with SS individuals without it. Indeed, such a pattern was reported in 1983 by Mears and his colleagues, but the population samples studied were too small to draw definitive conclusions. Stronger evidence of a survival advantage of alpha-thalassemia was found by examining its incidence among individuals in the three African population groups. In this case Pagnier and her colleagues found a frequency of alpha-thalassemia in the Senegal group of SS individuals similar to the general Sengalese population, whereas the SS individuals from the Niger River and Zaire River areas had a frequency of alpha-thalassemia about twice the level typical of these regions. Presumably, the SS individuals with the milder Senegalese form of sickle cell anemia (due to the moderating effect of relatively high levels of hemoglobin F) derive less survival benefit due to the presence of alpha-thalassemia than the SS individuals from other parts of Africa with relatively low fetal hemoglobin levels.[14]

It is clear that a complete understanding of sickle cell anemia will require careful examination of the influences arising from these and other genetic factors. For example, a particularly mild form of sickle cell anemia found in Saudi Arabia appears to be due to elevated levels of fetal hemoglobin. While elevated fetal hemoglobin levels do not occur as widely as alpha-thalassemia among blacks, additional studies of the molecular basis of this condition could suggest further avenues for therapy at the level of genes. It is conceivable that at some future time prenatal testing for alpha-thalassemia-2 or other chromosomal markers that may be correlated with severity will be routinely conducted. These additional factors might make the decision whether to terminate a pregnancy for an SS fetus more easily reached. However, such trying decisions will continue to be complicated by the possibility that a treatment for sickle cell anemia will be developed in the coming years. Action directly on hemoglobin S or the red cell membrane, if not a gene-switching drug, appear to be the most promising avenues for reversing the symptoms of sickling, as the next chapter will show.

CHAPTER 8

THE SEARCH FOR ANTISICKLING AGENTS

If prenatal diagnosis of sickle cell anemia and selective abortion of affected fetuses become more commonplace, the number of homozygous SS individuals born in the United States and other medically advanced countries may diminish somewhat. But these strategies are not likely to reduce greatly the number of newborns with sickle cell anemia in the rest of the world. As medical care to combat the early effects of sickle cell anemia improves, we can expect to see augmented numbers of SS individuals in the population. The increase will be modest in the United States, where survival is already fairly high, but it is potentially very great in Africa. As a result of this larger population of SS survivors, there will be a pressing and ever-increasing need for an effective antisickling drug. Our society continues to have great faith in pharmacology's ability to create new drugs for major afflictions such as cancer. This faith is justified in large part by past progress. In the early part of this century, the average life expectancy in the United States and Western Europe was less than 45 years; but enormous reductions in infectious diseases through the use of antibiotics and vaccines, along with improvements in other areas of health care, including nutrition and sanitation, have increased life expectancy to over 70 in Western countries today.

In contrast with the diseases successfully attacked by modern drugs, sickle cell anemia poses a number of special problems that thwart efforts to find a definitive "cure." Because sickling involves inherited changes in hemoglobin, a protein present in the body in very large amounts, a cure would require genetic engineering that is still well beyond current technology. Therefore, we are left with the hope that the symptoms can be treated on a continuing basis to counter the most noxious features of the disease. Such treatment would involve maintaining the individuals on a drug that acts either on the genes, the hemoglobin, or some other aspect of cellular activity. Drugs that act at the level of DNA to stimulate synthesis of fetal hemoglobin are a potential route for therapy that is just beginning to be explored. About a decade ago efforts were begun to treat the symptoms by chemical agents that act directly on the hemoglobin S molecules; and more recently, agents that act on the membrane of sickling cells have also been investigated. Although the results have not generated an effective drug, valuable experience has been gained. It is these approaches that we will now consider.[1]

Before the structural details of hemoglobin S fibers were deduced, knowledge that sickling was triggered by the amino acid valine led Makio Murayama to propose that the interactions of hemoglobin S responsible for the self-association into fibers were largely hydrophobic, or "water-avoiding." As in an oil slick that floats on a body of water, hydrophobic substances tend to stick together, driven to associate by their insolubility in a watery environment. Since valine has strong hydrophobic properties, it was reasoned that substances which break up hydrophobic interactions might work to interfere with fiber formation by hemoglobin S and thereby reverse the sickling of cells. One such substance is urea, a very simple organic molecule found in urine, where it serves to excrete nitrogen waste.[2]

In the early 1970s patients were treated with urea by R. M. Nalbandian, with some success reported.[3] Unfortunately, subsequent double-blind studies (those in which two sets of patients are given either a placebo or the drug to be tested, with neither the patient nor the attending physician aware of the true nature of the material administered) found no benefits for urea in relieving the crises of sickle cell anemia. Such carefully controlled tests are especially important for sickle cell crises, since patients will generally recover in several days even in the absence of specific treatment.

During the time of optimism that urea might provide relief against sickling, an important insight into its possible mode of action was made by Anthony Cerami and James Manning.[4] They noted that urea slowly breaks down to form small amounts of cyanate, a chemical known to react with proteins. Therefore, they reasoned, the small amounts of cyanate present in urea might be responsible for whatever benefits urea treatment provided. In experiments with isolated sickle cells treated with cyanate, they were able to demonstrate that cyanate did appreciably lessen the extent of sickling. Since reactions of cyanate with hemoglobin interfere with certain interactions that stabilize the T state, the allosteric transition is shifted in favor of the R state (see Chapter 5). As a result, the hemoglobin binds oxygen more tightly, fewer molecules of hemoglobin are in the T state at any moment, and there is a reduction in the formation of the fibers responsible for sickling.

These results spurred considerable hope that a treatment for sickling might be at hand, and the testing of cyanate quickly passed to clinical trials with human subjects. Unfortunately, severe side effects on the nervous systems of patients soon became apparent, and the studies were terminated. Nevertheless, hope was held out that cyanate might still be a useful treatment for sickle cell patients if blood samples were first removed from their bodies. The process of drawing blood samples, treating the red cells, removing excess cyanate, and returning the cells to the body (extracorporeal administration of the drug) has been followed in a number of trials with cyanate, but the effects on sickling have not been encouraging. Apparently, cyanate is less effective in preventing crises than had been expected from the laboratory tests with sickled cells. Even if it had been more successful in trials, the extracorporeal method of treatment would have been cumbersome and impractical for many medical centers, as well as relatively expensive. Therefore, cyanate has been abandoned as an antisickling agent for use in patients.[5]

In the last decade, dozens of other compounds have been suggested as possible antisickling agents and tested in the laboratory. A number of these act on the red cell membrane to alter the balance of ions and water in ways that may reduce sickling. Since sickling is stimulated by dehydration of red cells, drugs that help to rehydrate the cells could have beneficial effects. While the laboratory results on many potential antisickling agents have been modestly encouraging, few of the results have been sufficiently promising (or have involved chemicals that are sufficiently nontoxic) to warrant testing in patients. When clinical trials have been conducted, none of the effects in reducing the crises associated with sickle cell anemia were dramatic, with the latest drug tested, Cetiedil, found to give only slight relief for patients in crisis.[6]

At the present time no antisickling agent is routinely used to treat individuals with sickle cell anemia. A few moderately promising candidates are on the horizon, but many hurdles remain. Thus, in spite of our knowledge of virtually every aspect of sickling at the molecular level, it has not been possible to design an effective treatment. For most diseases that have been successfully treated with drugs, the relevant agents have been discovered by trial and error rather than rational design. But the massive drug screening programs that such an approach requires are not likely to be funded for sickle cell anemia, since the number of afflicted individuals is proportionately smaller than the number of cancer or heart disease victims, to take two examples. In addition, there are no animals with sickle cell disease that can be used for drug development. The cell sickling found in certain species of deer and other ungulates is promoted by oxygenation, not deoxygenation as in humans, and thus does not initiate the vicious cycle wherein sickling promotes deoxygenation which in turn promotes more sickling. Therefore, studying the effects of potential antisickling drugs in deer would not be useful. In the absence of an animal model or funds for massive screening, efforts to find antisickling agents has relied on testing red blood cells isolated from SS individuals or purified hemoglobin S, but as the case of cyanate makes clear, the limitations of such tests can be serious.

By far the greatest research activity has centered on chemical agents that interact directly with hemoglobin. Two types of compounds have been used: (1) compounds that bind reversibly without the formation of new covalent chemical bonds; and (2) compounds that bind irreversibly via the formation of a covalent bond with a portion of the hemoglobin S molecule. Most of the drugs used successfully to treat human diseases are of the first type, noncovalent; urea, itself incapable of forming covalent bonds with proteins, was originally believed to act in this way. The reaction postulated for cyanate was of the second type, covalent. The great advantage of covalent reactions is that the products of the reaction are permanent and can accumulate with relatively small doses of the agent. By contrast, the noncovalent agents must be supplied in relatively large amounts in order to maintain a sufficiently high concentration to bind to an appreciable fraction of the target molecules. A disadvantage of covalent agents is that they are often toxic, and undesirable side effects may be difficult to avoid, as was the case with cyanate.

Whether covalent or noncovalent, the goal for such agents is to prevent, reduce, or reverse the self-association of hemoglobin S molecules into fibers. These effects on fiber formation could take place either by a direct blockage of the intermolecular contacts responsible for stabilization of the fibers, or indirectly by increasing the affinity of hemoglobin for oxygen. Since it is predominantly the deoxygenated form (T state) of hemoglobin S that assembles into fibers, any increase in affinity of hemoglobin S for oxygen would reduce the fraction of molecules in the T state at partial saturations with oxygen and thereby reduce fiber formation. By shifting the oxygen binding curve to the left in the presence of the drug, more hemoglobin S molecules would remain oxygenated (and hence in the R state) at a particular oxygen pressure than in the absence of the drug.

Any antisickling drug that inhibits fiber formation will cause some left shifting of the oxygen binding curve, since the presence of fibers causes an excess shift to the right. However, a number of the antisickling compounds that have been tested to date act largely or entirely by this indirect mechanism of raising the affinity for oxygen without directly interrupting intermolecular contacts in the fibers. While a successful antisickling drug that acts only by raising the affinity of hemoglobin for oxygen is not out of the question, it would pose certain difficulties. For example, a patient treated with such a drug could experience a period of reduced (though not totally absent) sickling that would alleviate significantly the anemia normally associated with the disease. However, should the patient then experience a state of unusually low oxygen levels in the blood (as a consequence of vigorous exercise, for example) extensive sickling could occur and a more serious crisis could result—owing to the lessening of the anemia—than any that occurred before treatment. In addition, since the treated cells will tend to retain their oxygen, untreated cells will undergo more extensive deoxygenation and hence additional sickling. Therefore, a drug that acts by this indirect mechanism might show short-term results that were encouraging, but carry major risks in long-term treatment. Clearly, such subtleties greatly complicate the development of a successful antisickling agent.

Of the numerous compounds that have been tested for their reactions with hemoglobin, the covalent compounds have been characterized more fully in terms of their sites of reactivity on the hemoglobin S molecule, although information for noncovalent reagents has also recently begun to emerge from studies by x-ray crystallography. Two approaches have been taken in these studies: (1) a target is selected and then reagents are tailored to improve their reactivity with the target, or (2) reagents that show some antisickling properties are identified and then modified to improve their antisickling abilities, often without the researcher's knowing the specific site of reactivity.

In general, the specific target for chemical modification of a protein is the molecular pocket that tightly binds a small metabolite or substrate, since only the precise molecular architecture of such an "active site" has the conformational detail necessary for specificity. The regions of the hemoglobin S surface that participate in the various intermolecular contacts of the sickle helix, as presented in Figures 6.5–6.7, show no obvious distinguishing features to qualify them as specific targets. The fact that contacts form only at extremely high concentrations of hemoglobin is an indication that they are generally very weak and for this reason likely to lack specificity. The active site for the primary function of the hemoglobin molecule is the heme-binding pocket, but it is not a suitable target because heme binds so tightly to the globin chains that it effectively blocks the action of any other agents at this site.

Hemoglobin also possesses a specific binding pocket for the effector molecule 2,3-diphosphoglycerate (DPG), and the pocket, which lies between the beta chains (as illustrated in Figure 5.2), has the properties of an active site. One line of research that has exploited this site was developed by studying aspirin and various aspirin derivatives. As the research evolved, compounds were developed with a high degree of specificity for the DPG site, especially a double aspirin derivative (or diaspirin) that reacts with both beta chains at the positions that normally bind DPG. A crosslink is formed between the beta-82 lysine residues, causing a slight retraction of the nearby "receptor" pocket involving the beta-85 phenylalanine that binds the critical beta-6 valine residue of an adjacent hemoglobin S molecule. This retraction presumably accounts for weakened intermolecular interactions, resulting in diminished fiber formation and sickling. For the hemoglobin molecules reacted with the diaspirin, DPG can no longer be bound. Compounds of this type have potential as specific antisickling agents, although by blocking DPG binding they produce an increased affinity of hemoglobin for oxygen and this may complicate their utility. Such molecules have not advanced as antisickling agents beyond the preliminary screening stage.[7]

One other natural target on the hemoglobin molecule is the reactive sulfur atom of one of the amino acids containing sulfur, cysteine. Hemoglobin possesses three pairs of cysteine residues, but only the pair occurring at the beta-93 positions reacts readily with added chemical agents. Many such compounds, called thiol reagents, react with these cysteine residues, particularly in the oxygenated conformation (R state) of hemoglobin. Antisickling effects of thiol reagents have been described in a number of laboratories; Garel and her coworkers characterized 21 thiol reagents, many of which have antisickling properties.[8] In most cases, the antisickling effects of thiol reagents are related to an increase in the affinity of hemoglobin for oxygen, although in some cases a direct inhibition of fiber formation also occurs, perhaps related to a distortion of the receptor pocket on each hemoglobin S molecule that binds the beta-6 valine of the adjacent molecule across the double strand. For this receptor site the key residues— beta-85 phenylalanine and beta-88 leucine—occur only a few turns away from the beta-93 cysteine position in the same stretch of alpha helix. While the beta-93 represents a highly specific target on the hemoglobin molecule for thiol reagents, other proteins of the body might also react well with any particular thiol reagent, leading to possible toxicity. Another problem for thiol reagents concerns the reactive cysteine of the abundant serum albumin protein, which may trap a large fraction of a reagent before it enters the red cells. A third problem is that the bonds between thiol reagents and proteins are relatively labile.

Apart from these obvious targets, a number of sites have been discovered by the relatively specific reactivity of certain reagents. For example, glyceraldehyde reacts preferentially at the alpha-16 lysine residue to inhibit sickling. The lysine residue lies at the intermolecular contact along individual strands in the fibers. Nitrogen mustard reacts with histidine residues to inhibit sickling markedly. Although the extreme toxicity of nitrogen mustard severely limits its usefulness as an antisickling drug, whatever properties have led to the special reactivity may be exploited with other less toxic reagents. Other aldehydes with antisickling properties, as well as other types of covalent agents, that react with specific portions of the hemoglobin molecule have also been described, including a number of crosslinking agents and a known diuretic, ethacrynic acid.[9]

Fiber formation can also be inhibited by many agents that bind noncovalently, such as ethanol and other polar organic solvents, but the major effort in the development of noncovalent antisickling agents has focused on agents with a more complex structure. When a carbon atom has four different substituents attached to it, the resulting molecules can occur in two spatial configurations or forms that are related by a mirror image. Since pure solutions of each form rotate polarized light in opposite directions, the mirror image forms are called "stereoisomers." Much of the activity concerning noncovalent antisickling agents has involved stereospecific inhibitors, particularly amino acids, peptides, and related small molecules. For amino acids, the two stereoisomers are designated by D and L. Since proteins are made up entirely of amino acids in the L configuration, most compounds studied as antisickling agents are also of the L type. The dominant antisickling effect indicated by the studies of many peptides and amino acid derivatives is hydrophobicity, with one of the most nonpolar amino acids, L-phenylalanine (and L-phenylalanine-containing compounds), exhibiting relatively strong antisickling effects. Overall, improvements in the antisickling activity of compounds of the noncovalent class might lead to viable antisickling agents, but a major obstacle would be achieving suitable concentrations in the blood stream. Large amounts of the compounds would need to be ingested or injected to maintain a high concentration in the red cells, perhaps as much as a pound a day.[10]

One noncovalent compound of special interest is DBA, an analog of a natural product reported to have antisickling activity. It is believed to be the active ingredient of a "chewing stick" used in Africa that was suspected of providing some protection against sickling. The possibility of an antisickling agent derived from a natural product in use in Africa generated considerable excitement, but further studies with DBA have not been particularly encouraging.[11] Nevertheless, searching for a medicinal plant with antisickling properties remains a reasonable activity, particularly in view of suggestions that dietary factors may influence the properties of hemoglobin S. While we tend to associate many of the drugs currently in use for various diseases with the genius of laboratory scientists, the early successes in developing specific chemicals as drugs relied heavily on medicinal plants, beginning in the early 1800s with morphine and followed in the latter part of the same century by quinine and digitaline.

The history of quinine is especially relevant because of its connection with malaria. Quinine was discovered from extracts of the bark of a South American tree used to treat fevers. The bark made its first appearance in Europe in the 1600s, but it may well have been already in use among South American Indians for a very long time. According to tradition (although apocryphal on the basis of some sources), treatment with this medicine provided a spectacular cure of a certain Comptesse Del Chinchón, wife of the viceroy of Peru, who suffered from a severe fever that recurred every three days. Such a repeating pattern of fever is one of the signs of malaria. Her fame spread sufficiently that Linne, a century later, baptized the tree in question in her honor, with the designation *Cinchona.* The cinchona bark was brought in large quantities to Rome by the Jesuits and the bitter-tasting extract produced from the bark achieved a wide renown in Europe for its curative powers.

A proper scientific description of the cinchona tree in its habitat involved a number of efforts (and mishaps) before being completed in the early nineteenth century. Soon afterward, Joseph Pelletier and Joseph Caventou isolated quinine. Large-scale production followed, although not without risk of making the trees extinct. Therefore, tree farms of cinchona were attempted by the

Dutch in Java and by the English in India, but both produced trees with very low levels of quinine. Evidently, the Peru Indians had never permitted the Europeans to know exactly which species of cinchona tree was the most effective. Finally, an Englishman named Ledger obtained growths from the efficient species, known as *Cinchona ledgeriana,* and the Dutch succeeded in establishing farms in Java. Production on the eve of World War II achieved an annual level of 1,500 tons. The capture of Java by the Japanese during World War II interrupted the supply of quinine, and efforts to develop artificial substitutes were launched. A number of successful synthetic antimalarials, such as chloraquine, have been widely used since that time. However, as *Plasmodium* strains have become increasingly resistant to these new products, quinine use has been renewed, especially in Southeast Asia.[12]

The quinine story illustrates the fact that an effective drug can be discovered before the disease it combats is characterized. Quinine was used in treating fevers before malaria was identified as a disease caused by parasites transmitted by mosquitos. Indeed, the name "malaria" derives from the Italian term for the "bad air" that was believed to arise from swamps and cause the disease. By analogy, it remains possible that an African society has discovered a natural treatment for the symptoms of sickle cell anemia in total ignorance of sickling cells. Therefore, additional field work in Africa should be attempted to pursue this possibility. It is ironic that a natural antimalarial was discovered in South America, but not in Africa. If early African societies had discovered a plant agent effective against malaria, the sickle mutation might not have had a selective advantage and sickle cell anemia might not be a major problem today. Indeed, the presence of an antimalarial plant in South America may explain the very low levels of hemoglobin pathology on that continent today.

Historical records of medicinal uses of plants have been found as far back as ancient Babylon, Egypt, and China. But despite the prodigious powers of traditional societies for naming the diversity of plants around them and for formulating ingenious uses, relatively few successful modern products have been derived from this vast store of knowledge and tradition. One reason is that in traditional societies, the consumption of natural medicines is usually linked to a series of ritual acts within which the role of the plant products may be as much symbolic as physiological. As a result, a dilemma is squarely posed concerning the value of information from traditional sources. As noted by one specialist, J.-M. Pelt,

> Such is the force, but also the weakness of the empiricism and life in the heart of traditional societies: a precise organization, highly codified; unshakable traditions, solidly anchored, that provide a strong sense of security—these elements interpret illness and integrate death in a system of coherent values uniformly accepted by all members of the society. However, at the same time, any false beliefs or erroneous interpretations are perpetuated from generation to generation, as sources of suffering. Hence, a selection must be imposed. Reject everything as a block—this would deprive us of novel sources of discovery. Condemn the practices for the reason that they are not "scientific"—this would be the most unscientific attitude of all. Nevertheless, to accept everything—this would constitute a wish to return to the past, as in a utopian dream.[13]

The heritage of traditional medicine is thus greatly complicated by the dual role of plants as symbols and as physical agents. This is especially true in Africa, where illness is traditionally believed to be caused by spiritual forces and the power of a drug is held to depend more on the power of the traditional doctor or healer than on the intrinsic potency of the drug. An additional difficulty is the "personalization" of illness. Since in the African tradition each individual is rendered ill by a particular set of forces, the medicines prescribed may be vastly different even for similar symptoms. Another complication may arise concerning dose, since the recommendations of a traditional healer may vary widely, sometimes with unanticipated results. As reported by Aujoulat for the practitioners of Cameroon, accidents tend not to discredit the drug or the healer, but are explained by the notion that "the medicine was too strong for the patient." Thus, the healer may warn the patient that "the medicines may be too strong," but this apparently does not generally discourage the patient.[14]

In the development of the European tradition of medicines from plants, a key step was Galen's recognition in the second century of the importance of dose. Earlier authorities appeared indifferent to dose, and in the biblical tradition medicinal plants have played only a very minor role. The Old Testament placed the outcome of adversity or illness in the hands of an all-powerful divinity, so little need appeared to exist for mere medicines. Thus, according to Meyer, the only reference to medicinal uses of plants in the Old Testament concerns the promotion of virility attributed to mandrake. Healing traditions involving plants in Christian times were largely in the hands of monasteries, and even they were subjected periodically to reforms aimed at discontinuing the practices. It is likely that the garden attended to by Mendel had its origins in the monastic tradition of healing through the use of plants.

Any evaluation of the power of a particular natural product is even further complicated by the fact that in traditional societies the patient is generally given a mixture of five or six different plants. Interestingly, a similar strategy might emerge concerning modern drugs for sickle cell anemia. The amount of hemoglobin that must be modified is so great (up to two pounds of this protein circulate in the blood) that any one antisickling drug in the concentrations needed might be too toxic. The usual pharmacological requirements for specificity and safety would be hard to meet at the necessary doses, even for a compound as widely used as aspirin. However, satisfactory results might be achieved with a mixture of several drugs at more modest concentrations.

Aspirin is another medicine with ancient roots. It was first extracted from the bark of willow trees, in the quest for a fever-reducing agent. Willow bark, like cinchona bark, produces an extract with a bitter taste. According to the traditional argument, the successful growth of willow trees in wet areas indicated a power to overcome fever that arose from wet feet. In addition, the tree's ability to relieve joint stiffness was suggested by the flexibility of the branches. As silly as these arguments appear today, they were presented in all seriousness to the Royal Society of London in 1763. In spite of any spurious arguments about willow trees, an active ingredient, named salicine, was eventually isolated from willow bark. Salicylic aldehyde was also isolated from the plant meadowsweet (*Spiraea ulmaria*) and was later oxidized to salicylic acid. An acetylated derivative, acetylsalicylic acid, was synthesized by a chemist working for the Bayer Pharmaceutical Company, and the success of aspirin was launched. The name "aspirin" was coined from "a" for "acetylated," plus "spir" for the species *Spiraea* from which part of it had been obtained.[15]

While aspirin has an impressive ability to lower fever and relieve pain, its mode of action remains poorly understood. A number of authorities maintain that if aspirin had been discovered for the first time only recently, it would probably be rejected by the Food and Drug Administration because of certain side effects (such as stomach irritation) and difficulties in quantitating its activity. If aspirin would have such difficulties today, we can imagine the problems that would face an antisickling agent that must also be given in large doses. Promising compounds that work well as antisickling agents in laboratory tests with sickled cells will face difficult hurdles of safety and efficacy before entering into general usage, particularly since individuals with sickle cell anemia would often need to be maintained on the drug for long periods of time.

In summary, despite a considerable history of research on agents that inhibit sickling, strong candidates for routine use have not yet emerged. Therefore, novel approaches to treating sickle cell anemia should also be considered, particularly at the level of the red cell membrane and, as discussed in Chapter 7, the beta-globin gene. For example, a targeted delivery system, in which antisickling drugs are encapsulated in membranes that fuse specifically with red blood cells, might reduce the necessary dose of drugs acting on hemoglobin. Many steps remain to be worked out before such a system could be implemented, but preliminary studies have been sufficiently promising to warrant continued research. Drugs that act on certain secondary effects of sickling might also prove to be useful. One consequence of sickling appears to be that cells become "sticky," and this stickiness may be an important element in producing the clinical symptoms of sickle cell anemia. Hebbel and others have reported that when red cells are placed in contact with endothelial cells (as occur in the lining of blood vessels) that have been cultured in the laboratory, the red cells from SS individuals stick to the endothelial cells more strongly than red cells from AA individuals. Therefore, another avenue to explore for antisickling agents involves drugs that act directly on this enhanced adhesion of sickled cells to blood vessel walls.[16]

Stickiness is just one manifestation of sickling at the membrane level. Membranes are composed of sheets of phospholipids, molecules with polar "heads" and nonpolar "tails." Two sheets, tails together, form the lipid bilayer that envelops all cells. Imbedded in the phospholipids are the various proteins responsible for transport across the membrane. Several classes of phospholipids can be distinguished, depending on the nature of the compound that makes up the "head": choline in the phospholipid phosphatidyl-choline (abbreviated PC); ethanolamine in PE; and serine in PS. In normal red cells, most of the PC is in the outer layer of the membrane bilayer, while PE and PS reside in the inner layer. Among the changes in the red cell membrane found to accompany sickling is a destabilization of the membrane lipid bilayer, such that PE and PS become accessible on the outside. These findings may be related to the pinching off of small membrane vesicles (called "spicules") that is known to occur at the pointed tips of sickled cells. These changes at the surface of sickled cells, including changes in the properties or distribution of membrane proteins, may contribute to their heightened stickiness; thus, a drug that could moderate these effects might reduce some symptoms of sickle cell anemia. Conceivably, beneficial effects could be achieved with much smaller quantities of such a drug than would be necessary for a drug that modifies hemoglobin, since the number of molecules on the surface of a red cell is far smaller than the number of hemoglobin molecules within the cell.[17] For most sickled cells, the membrane is not permanently distorted, since partial lysis will restore the membrane to its oval shape (Fig. 8.1).

Another possible strategy for attacking sickling at a point where lower levels of a drug would be required concerns the concentration of 2,3-DPG. This small molecule of the red cell stabilizes the T state of hemoglobin, as was shown in Figure 5.2, and promotes fiber formation. Therefore, a treatment that specifically lowered 2,3-DPG levels in the red cells of homozygous SS individuals might improve their condition. Since DPG is formed by the enzyme DPG mutase, which occurs in the red cell at concentrations thousands of times lower than hemoglobin, relatively small amounts of a suitable drug that inhibited the enzyme could have a significant effect. However, there is currently insufficient information concerning the properties of the mutase to indicate what kind of compound could act as such an anti-DPG (and thus anti-sickling) drug by inhibiting the mutase.

Overall, on the basis of the experience with a number of categories of antisickling agents, the next generation of antisickling agents developed may reasonably be expected to achieve improved efficacies, perhaps suitable for therapeutic use. What form such agents will take is not yet clear, and ample opportunities re-

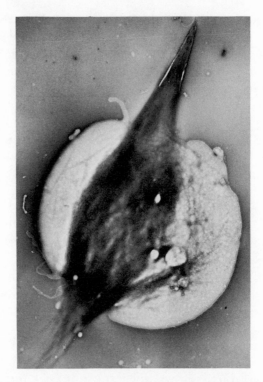

Figure 8.1. Electron micrograph of partially lysed sickled cell. Lysis by negative stain at the tips of the cell released the membrane to return to its normal oval shape, while the bundles of fibers remained in their sicklelike arrangement.

main for creative medicinal chemistry to be applied. With the use of powerful computers, the possibility exists to "test" compounds with computer models based on a study of the atomic structure and energetics of the complete hemoglobin molecule in combination with the candidate drug. Proposed compounds that appear to be especially promising could then be tested directly with sickled cells. Such computer-aided drug design has recently been widely discussed for a number of diseases involving protein molecules of known structure, and hemoglobin would appear to be an ideal candidate. My colleagues and I have initiated such efforts for compounds of the thiol class that react with the beta-93 cysteine. Initial efforts representing the region of this residue alone and after reaction with a cyclic thiol compound are presented in Figure 8.2. For the relatively bulky thiopyridine derivative of

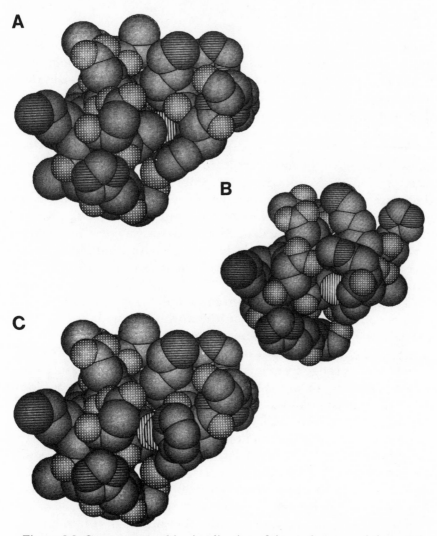

Figure 8.2. Computer graphic visualization of the pocket around the reactive cysteine, beta 93. (A) The pocket for the hemoglobin molecule in the R state with the reactive thiol group of the cysteine indicated by vertical stippling. Other types of atoms are indicated by horizontal stippling for nitrogen, cross hatching for oxygen, and solid gray scales for carbon. (B) The same residues as in (A), but for the T state of hemoglobin in which the 5-membered ring of the C-terminal histidine forms a "salt bridge" with the aspartic acid next to the cysteine; this salt bridge contributes to the stabilization of the T state. (C) Hemoglobin in the R state reacted with a model antisickling drug (2-thiopyridine) composed of a thiol group and a six-membered ring with one nitrogen atom. Drugs of this type can act both to raise oxygen affinity, by blocking the salt bridge seen in (B), and to perturb contacts between molecules in the fibers.

hemoglobin illustrated in the figure, two types of effects are suggested by the computer modeling: disturbing the salt bridge between aspartate beta-93 and histidine beta-146 that stabilizes the T state; and perturbing the region around the cysteine beta-93 that participates in intermolecular contacts within the sickle helix.

Time will tell which of the various approaches discussed in this chapter will have the most success in reversing the devastating effects of sickling. While the basic problems remain formidable, there are enough routes showing some promise that we can express guarded optimism for the appearance in the coming years of an effective antisickling drug. Such a development would mark yet another impact of the sickle cell upon the human experience—in this case, stimulating one of the first major achievements in rational drug design.

The topics which have been prompted by a consideration of the sickled cell make it clear that the metaphor with which we started—the grain of sand whose contemplation reveals the universe—was not so great an exaggeration. The dimensions applied to sickled cells range from mere angstroms needed to measure the valine at position six of the beta chains of hemoglobin responsible for sickling, to thousands of miles needed to measure the spread of the sickle mutation in various societies. The sickled cell has also pointed us toward considerations of the extremes of form, from the regularities of helices to the irregularities of birth defects, and the extremes of human experience, from the logic of the scientific approach to the intuitive formulations of myth. In exploring just one aspect of the human experience, a relatively simple genetic disease, we have been led to consider the similarity of humans to their primate relatives and the integration of living organisms within the molecular world. If we consider time, sickled cells point us toward both the fractions of a second sufficient to provoke sickling of a single cell, and the centuries required for the rise of the sickle mutation to its current incidence in human populations. But even centuries represent a remarkably short period of time for a species to progress from hunting and gathering to manipulating its environment and its own chemical constituents.

1. THE SICKLE OF AFRICA

1. The molecular and cellular aspects of sickling have been described in a number of monographs; among the more recent are the books by Bunn et al. (1977); Caughey (1978); Siegler (1981); Beuzard et al. (1984); Bunn and Forget (1985); Serjeant (1985).

2. Throughout this book the spelling "Igbo" is used, since it is favored by most recent authors, although earlier writers regularly used the spelling "Ibo."

3. The report by Herrick (1910) concerning sickled cells was a major accomplishment. Herrick is also credited with one of the first reports of a heart attack.

4. The classification of African languages into four phyla refers to the description of Joseph Greenberg (1955), which has been largely accepted by African linguists. The four classes are Afro-Asiatic (including Hausa, Arabic, Hebrew, and ancient Egyptian); Niger-Congo-Kordofian, Nilo-Saharan, and Khosian. Languages that were transcribed in Arabic script before the contacts with Europeans are discussed by Alexandre (1981).

5. Welmers (1973), p. 79. The example which follows is from the same book, p. 82. Tones are of course essential in Chinese, where the same sound can have up to four different meanings in the Beijing dialect and up to nine in the Cantonese dialect; see E. Glahn in Toynbee (1973).

6. Bowen (1964), p. 16. For a summary of writings of the first European visitors, see Hibbert (1982).

7. Example from Maquet (1981).

8. The quote is from I. Karp (Karp and Bird, 1980). Concerning the difference between French and English scholars, see Turner (1965).

9. The population density maximum was reported by Uchenda (1965).

10. Lévi-Strauss (1966), p. 14. Details of the excavations can be found in Shaw (1978).

11. Jacob (1982), pp. 33–34.

12. The information concerning Igbo death concepts is from Noon (1942).

13. Isichei (1976), pp. 26–27.

14. The early missionaries' reports are summarized by Henderson (1972).

15. Achebe (1969), pp. 74–75.

2. EVOLUTION AND HEMOGLOBIN

1. Zuckerkandl and Pauling (1962).

2. Wilson et al. (1971) and Goodman et al. (1983); see also Dickerson and Geis (1983).

3. For additional discussions of primate evolution see: Sarich and Wilson (1967), Coppens (1983), and Pilbeam (1984); and for the latter stages: Ciochon and Corruccini (1983) and Smith and Spencer (1984).

4. The arguments in favor of a stronger human–gorilla similarity are presented by Miller (1977), and a stronger human–orangutan similarity by Schwartz (1984).

5. For behavioral studies, see Goodall et al. (1979) and Fossey (1979). References on chimpanzee cannibalism include Bygott (1972) and Itani (1982).

6. Hemoglobin sequences are from Goodman et al. (1983). Proteins that are identical for humans and chimpanzees include fibrinopeptides A and B and cytochrome c; one difference exists for myoglobin and hemoglobin delta chains.

The following terms are applied to the classification of human beings—superfamily: Hominoidea; family: Hominidae; subfamily: Homininae; genus: *Homo;* species: *Homo sapiens;* subspecies: *Homo sapiens sapiens.*

7. See Coppens (1983); Pilbeam (1984); Ciochon and Corruccini (1983); and Smith and Spencer (1984).

8. *Homo habilis* was described by Leaky et al. (1964).

9. Analysis of nine globins: Lesk and Chothia (1980).

10. For a more complete discussion of punctuated evolution, see Gould (1982).

11. Parallel evolution and horses are discussed in A. Leroi-Gourhan (1983).

12. For a careful analysis of DNA differences for humans, chimpanzees, gorillas, orangutans, and gibbons, see Sibley and Ahlquist (1984).

13. Diamond (1984).

14. Geschwind (1974), pp. 454–456.

15. Translated by the author from Coppens (1983), p. 119.

3. THE MICROEVOLUTION OF SICKLING

1. For additional information on the early history of hemoglobin see Edsall (1972).

2. Stent and Calendar (1978), p. 7.

3. Statistics on the sickle mutation indicating inheritance according to principles of Mendel were originally summarized by Neel (1949).

4. The conclusion concerning malaria fatality among children in Nigeria is from Attah and Ejekam (1974).

5. General information on the clinical manifestations of sickle cell anemia from Bunn et al. (1977); concerning dactylitis, see Serjeant and Ashcroft (1971). Additional information available from the Natural History Study conducted by the Sickle Cell Branch, National Institutes of Health (Bethesda, Maryland).

6. Information on infections in sickle cell disease for patients in the United States is from Overturf and Powers (1981); comparisons with infections in Ghana are from Ringelhann (1973).

7. The mathematical model for calculation of factors influencing frequency of the sickle mutation in the Igbo population and similar groups is based on the equations for balanced polymorphism of Cavalli-Sforza and Bodmer (1971). In their formulation, the terms Fitness (AA) and Fitness (SS) are represented as $(1 - s)$ and $(1 - t)$, respectively. The incidence of the S mutation is expressed as q, defined as one-half of the frequency of AS individuals plus twice the frequency of SS individuals. The equation for the relationship used to obtain the data in the table is $q = s/(s + t)$. The equation can be derived from the following considerations: We define p and q as the frequencies of the A and S genes, respectively (where $p = 1 - q$). Hence, the probability for an individual to be AA is p^2. This probability reflects the necessity for receipt of the A gene from the father (probability p), as well as from the mother (probability p). Similarly, the probability for an SS individual is q^2, while the probability of an AS individual is $1 - p^2 - q^2$. We may also define the relative incidence of the AS individuals as one and the incidences of AA and SS individuals as $1 - s$ and $1 - t$, respectively. According to the definitions of s and t, selection will eliminate AA individuals with a probability s and SS individuals with a probability t, to give weighted probabilities of elimination for the entire population in question of sp^2 and tq^2, respectively. Since the population is assumed to be at equilibrium, the ratio p/q is determined by the respective eliminations: $p/q = sp^2/tq^2$. Therefore, $sp = tq$, or $s(1 - q) = tq$, and solving for q, we obtain the relationship sought, $q = s/(s + t)$. The AS percentage of 25% for the Igbos is from Lehmann and Nwokolo (1959).

8. The report of malaria infection with AA and AS volunteers is from Allison (1954); see also Allison (1964). Results indicating less difference of AA and AS individuals with respect to malaria are presented by Jackson (1981).

9. For information on the population of Africa 2,000 years ago, see McEvedy (1980), p. 36.

10. For information on migrations in African history, see Fage (1979) and Livingstone (1976).

11. Herskovits (1958).

12. Konotey-Ahulu (1973), p. 36.

13. Information on Chief Onyeama is from the biography by his grandson (Onyeama, 1982). The experiments concerning effects of sickle hemoglobin on the growth of malaria parasites in red cells are described by Friedman and Trager (1981).

14. The general data on slavery are from Oliver and Crowder (1981). A history of the Igbo during the slave-trade period can be found in Isichei (1976).

15. Quotation on "Eboes" is from B. Edwards (1794), a text located in the Cornell University Rare Book collection. Other details are found in Herskovits (1958). On the Yoruba, see Thompson (1983).

16. List of slave names is from Puckett (1975), and translations of Igbo

names are from Njoko (1978). Other comments on Igbo manifestations in the New World are found in Paterson (1967).

17. Experiments reporting the effect of cyanate on the growth of the malaria parasite *P. falciparum* are described by Nagel et al. (1980b). Jackson's ideas are presented in articles in press (1986) and in preparation.

18. Durham's analysis of the sickle gene distribution is reported in his 1983 article. Additional information on new yam festivals is provided by Coursey and Coursey (1971).

19. The term "thalassemia" means literally illness of the sea, related presumably to the promoting of the development of malaria-bearing mosquitos in relatively wet regions near the sea, with the corresponding selection of the beta-thalassemia mutation that provided some resistance to malaria. When heterozygous individuals for beta-thalassemia reached significant levels, the severely ill homozygous individuals began to appear, naturally in regions near the sea, thus accounting for the origin of the name. For details concerning the origin of the deficiency in glucose-6-phosphate dehydrogenase, see Huheey and Martin (1976) and Golenser et al. (1983). Results concerning the low oxygen levels needed for growth of *Plasmodium falciparum* in red blood cells are presented by Trager and Jensen (1976).

20. A general discussion of toxic compounds of diet is presented by Ames (1983). Indications that increased oxidation may be a consequence of sickling in red cells are provided by Das and Nair (1980) concerning levels of glutathione, peroxidase, catalase and malonyldialdehyde; Hebbel et al. (1982) concerning peroxide and other reactive forms of oxygen; Chiu and Lubin (1979) concerning alpha-tocopherol (vitamin E).

4. AFRICAN REPEATER CHILDREN

1. African concepts of ancestry and reincarnation are closely related to family structure in different societies. In general, patrilinear societies predominate; Mair (1960) reports 83% patrilinear and 17% matrilinear for 90 African societies characterized. For a more extensive discussion of specific aspects of belief among the Igbo concerning reincarnation, see Webb (1981).

2. Quotes concerning *ogbanje* from Okonji (1970), p. 1.

3. The quote concerning *ogbanje* and sickle cell disease is from Nwokolo (1960).

4. The article by James Onwubalili stressing the link between *ogbanje* and sickle cell anemia was published in the August 27, 1983, issue of the *Lancet*. A letter summarizing the poor correlation found for the Awgu children was published by S. Edelstein and I. Stevenson in the issue of November 12, 1983, and Onwubalili's letter of reply was published in the issue of December 7, 1983.

5. The information concerning dactylitis is from Bunn et al. (1977), pp. 255-256.

6. The list of terms comes from Konotey-Ahulu (1973); the Krobo tribe family is mentioned in Konotey-Ahulu (1974).

7. Bascom (1969), p. 74.

8. Soyinka (1981), pp. 15–16.

9. The quotation concerning the Igbo is from Ottenberg (1959), p. 130.

10. The quotation concerning the Azande is from Evans-Pritchard (1935), pp. 418–419.

11. For *àbikú* names, see Verger (1968).

12. Talbot (1967), p. 151; Verger (1968).

13. Abrahamsson (1951), p. 7; see also Frazer (1913).

14. Collomb (1973), p. 447.

15. Diebolt and Linhard (1969).

16. One of the early reports of repeater children from West Africa can be found in Charles Monteil's study of the Bambara, a large ethnic group centered in what now is Mali. Discussing the Bambara's belief in a projected shadow or double, called *dya*, Monteil (1924, pp. 120–121) notes that they used marking of cadavers to provide what was for them irrefutable proof of the return of children and other deceased relatives.

> It appears that to the *dya* is assigned the principal role in this 'return' (*sagi*), or coming back to life which is one of the firmest beliefs of the Bambara. After death, the *dya* reincarnates in the same family; some Bambara claim to have irrefutable proof of this fact. Is not a certain newborn child displaying a particular anatomical detail that was characteristic of a certain deceased person the proof that the deceased person wished to manifest his or her reincarnation by that sign? For children that die at an early age, a mark or specific mutilation is made on the body—a fracture of a finger, for example. If an infant is later born into the same family with a deformation that corresponds to the one made on the little cadaver, the conclusion is made that the deceased child has 'returned' and one says 'a sagira': 'he has come again'. [trans. au.]

Parrinder (1951) notes that among the Bambara a succeeding child born to the same mother with such identifying marks is often given a "shameful" name, either to make it ashamed of leaving the parents too soon or else to deceive other spirits into believing that it is worthless. The Mossi of Upper Volta give the name *yamba*, meaning "slave," to a child born after the deaths of several previous siblings. Then a neighbor pretends to buy the "slave" by giving money to the father, so that this claim of ownership will serve to prevent the infant from dying.

Another early report concerning peoples in the region now occupied by Ghana describes other subtle marking practices (Cardinall, 1920, pp. 66–67):

> If a child dies soon after birth, and the next one is of the same sex, it is believed that the dead child has returned . . . To recognize the dead [relative] in a new-born infant there are many signs. The most common are as follows: On the death of an infant the grave-diggers make a small mark with ashes on his cheek or forehead, and when the child is born again he will have the same mark on his forehead or cheek. Others, instead of marking the child with ashes, fold his little finger, and when he is re-born his little finger is bent.

A modern study of the LoDagaa of northwest Ghana reveals the persistence of such practices (Goody, 1962, p. 150):

> A child whose elder sibling has died is believed to be that elder sibling ... He is known as *tshaakuor* or *lewa*, 'one who comes back', is called by the special personal name of Der, or Yuora in the case of a girl, and is usually marked on the cheek with a cut so that he can be identified if he dies and returns again yet a third time. Sometimes the gravediggers will make a series of cuts on the corpse of such a child ... Then when the same mother bears again, the women who first bathe the newborn child look for evidence of such marks, and if they discern any, exclaim: 'He's come back! He's come back!' (*o le ba wa*). The intended effect of such cries is to shame (*yongna vii*) the errant child into staying on this earth; for it is thought that if he knows that others are aware of what he is about, he will no longer plague the mother.

In other reports concerning Ghana, Verger (1968) notes that the Fanti call repeater children *kossamah,* and Debrunner (1959), p. 43, cites the Akan tradition of giving a special name to the mother of repeater children: *awo-ma-wu,* which he defines as "one who brings forth children for death, meaning the children will all die prematurely in infancy."

Another recent report discusses "repeater children" of the Ijaw in the heart of the Niger Delta (Leis, 1982, pp. 156–157):

> If parents have experienced several infant deaths, one after another, they usually suspect that the same child is coming to them each time ... In an attempt to let the child know that he should not come back again if he intends dying once more or that he should remain living the next time he is born, the father will take the body to the forest, chop it into pieces and bury the remains in separate deep graves ... I was told of one little boy, about three years old at the time, who complained to his mother one day that he had really been hurt that time his father had cut him into pieces. His mother then admitted that they had indeed disposed of the body of a baby born sometime before the boy. I might add that the mother had not considered that the little boy had heard the tale elsewhere and was simply repeating it with his own embellishment; his comment was taken as evidence that a young child can remember a former existence.

This report indicates that the belief in repeater children can be reinforced by statements of children indicating knowledge of a past life (see Stevenson, 1983), as well as from physical features alleged to correspond to marks made previously on a cadaver. Brief note of such practices among other ethnic groups also has been published (Thomas and Luneau, 1977, p. 280):

> If a woman gives birth several times to a stillborn, one thinks immediately of the vengance of an ancestor. That is why the Diola [Senegal] mutilate the cadaver so that the ancestor so marked will not dare to reincarnate ... The Agni [Ivory Coast] believe that children that die have departed the spirit world surreptitiously in order to observe events

among the living or obtain a favor; then they run back to the *eblo*. In an effort to cure them, so that they remain on earth, eventually their ear is pierced to break the cycle of reincarnations. [trans. au.]

17. Information concerning Zaire is taken from Torday and Joyce (1910), pp. 125–126, and concerning Kenya from Hobley (1967), p. 159.

18. Livingston (1973).

19. Birth defects involving fingers have been described by Horton (1979). The early studies of ainhum have been reviewed by Kean and Tucker (1946), and more recent ideas on the causes of ainhum have been presented by Dent et al. (1981). The studies of ainhum concerning Africa are from Browne (1965).

20. Tylor (1958), p. 14; see also Delafosse (1908) and Malinowski (1954).

21. Paulme (1954), p. 142, trans. au.

22. Hobley (1967), p. 159.

23. Uchendu (1965), p. 6.

24. Parry (1932), pp. 398–399.

25. For additional details concerning "repeater child" from Thailand, see Stevenson (1983).

26. While explanations of the apparently mutilated hands of Gargas include loss of fingers due to frostbite or disguising of intact fingers to give the appearance of shortening as some kind of code (a view favored by Leroi-Gourhan, 1967) the weight of the evidence, as stressed by Sahly (1966), would appear to favor deliberate mutilations, although for reasons that remain mysterious.

5. THE MOLECULAR PERSPECTIVE

1. Monod (1971), p. 170.

2. Monod et al. (1965).

3. The description of the altered mobility in electric fields for hemoglobin from sickled cells was described in Pauling et al. (1949). (In addition to a Nobel Prize in Chemistry in 1954, Pauling received the Nobel Prize in Peace in 1962 for his efforts to end atmospheric testing of nuclear weapons.)

Perutz and Mitchison (1950) observed that the S form of hemoglobin was much less soluble than the normal form, suggesting that it would assume an aggregated state.

4. The identification of valine at the site of the sickle mutation was reported by Ingram (1956).

5. Watson and Crick (1953).

6. See Wang et al. (1979) or, for more recent views, Marx (1985).

7. For the reintroduction of the Pauling model, see Koshland et al. (1966). For a more complete discussion of the distinctions between these formulations of cooperativity, see Edelstein (1975).

8. Changeux (1983), p. 200.

9. For the application of the model of R and T states to hemoglobin mutants and the Bohr effect, see Edelstein (1971).

10. For the original presentation of the alpha helix, see Pauling and Corey

(1950). The triple helix model for DNA is described in Pauling and Corey (1953).

11. Monod (1968).

6. THE SICKLE HELIX

1. For early references to the structure of the fibers of hemoglobin S, as revealed by electron microscopy, see Bessis et al. (1958); Stetson (1966); Bertles et al. (1970); and White (1974).

2. Dykes et al. (1978).

3. Additional details of the structure of the fibers, including the original evidence for the pairing of strands, can be found in Dykes et al. (1979). Reconstructions providing evidence for pairing of strands within intact fibers are presented by Rodgers et al. (1986).

4. Wishner et al. (1975).

5. Evidence concerning the various sites on the beta chains of hemoglobin that influence fiber formation is presented by Nagel et al. (1980a), including agreement between positions of mutations that influence sickling and amino acids that lie at intermolecular contacts in the crystals. Magdoff-Fairchild and Chua (1979) have studied the relationship of x-ray diffraction of fibers and crystals, calling attention to the similarities. Deductions concerning the differences between fibers and crystals and maps showing the surface of hemoglobin with the locations of amino acids that lie at contacts are reported by Edelstein (1981).

6. For studies of alpha chain mutants in combination with beta-S chains related to the positions of intermolecular contacts, see Benesch et al. (1971), Rhoda et al. (1983), and, in relation to missing strands, Crepeau et al. (1981). Alternative aggregates of hemoglobin S that do not appear to be related to the 14-strand sickle helix found in SS red cells have been studied by Finch et al. (1973); Adachi and Asakura (1981); and Potel et al. (1984); see also Makinen and Sigountos (1984).

7. Coletta et al. (1982) summarize the work on rates of red cell sickling. Promotion of fiber formation by deoxygenation was first appreciated by Hahn and Gillespie (1927) and Ham and Castle (1940).

8. For studies of cell density heterogeneity, see Fabry and Nagel (1982).

9. Homogeneous and heterogeneous nucleation are described by Ferrone et al. (1985).

10. Details on fan-shaped packing are from Edelstein and Crepeau (1979).

11. Noguchi and Schecheter (1985).

12. The malaria parasite interactions with sickle red cells are described by Friedman and Trager (1981).

7. CONFRONTING SICKLING AT THE GENES

1. Some progress toward genetic manipulation has recently been achieved by Williams and coworkers (1984) in introducing a bacterial gene into blood-forming cells that were then transplanted into irradiated mice. Efficient engraftment of the bacterial gene-containing cells was achieved. Simi-

lar principles could be used to remove marrow from homozygous SS individuals, transform the cells, and restore them to the individual, although the various problems associated with bone marrow transplants would still exist. Along similar lines, Gruber et al. (1985) have recently described gene transfer into human blood-forming cells using viruses to deliver the genes. A cure of sickle cell anemia has been reported for a patient treated for leukemia by a bone-marrow transplant; see Johnson et al. (1984).

2. See Charache et al. (1983) and Ley et al. (1983).

3. DNA sequencing methods are described in Gilbert (1981) and Sanger (1981).

4. For the first reports on introns in hemoglobin genes, see Jeffreys and Flavell (1977) and Tilghman et al. (1978).

5. The terms "intron" and "exon" were coined by Walter Gilbert. For the significance of introns, see Gilbert (1978; 1985). Function studies on portions of globin defined by individual exons are described by Craik et al. (1980).

6. The use of *Mst*II in the diagnosis of sickle mutation is described by Chang and Kan (1982) and by Orkin et al. (1982).

7. Application of CVS to sickle cell anemia was reported by Old et al. (1982) and Gossens et al. (1983).

8. Konotey-Ahulu (1982).

9. Alter (1981); for more recent statistics, see Alter (1984).

10. Kan and Dozy (1980).

11. Data on the distribution of hemoglobin C were reported by Lehmann and Nwokolo (1959).

12. Evidence for more than two origins of the sickle mutation was presented by Pagnier et al. (1984). Some general observations on the use of hemoglobins in historical research have been presented by Bernard (1983). The report of higher F levels with the Senegalese pattern of sickle cell anemia is by Nagel et al. (1985).

13. The initial reports of slightly less severe sickle cell anemia when accompanied by alpha-thalassemia were by Embury et al. (1982) and Higgs et al. (1982). However, the recent report of Steinberg et al. (1984) indicates that less effect of alpha-thalassemia may occur than initially suspected, especially for American patients. Diseases related to sickle cell anemia but with markedly milder symptoms occur when the S gene is present in a heterozygous relationship with beta-thalassemia to give a condition known as S/Beta-thal, or with hemoglobin C to give SC disease (see Bunn et al., 1977; 1982).

14. Data on the frequency of alpha-thalessemia with age in sickle cell anemia patients is reported by Mears et al. (1983) and for the Senegal, Benin, and Central Africa populations by Pagnier et al. (1984).

8. THE SEARCH FOR ANTISICKLING AGENTS

1. This chapter is based on a recent review of antisickling agents (Edelstein, 1985).

2. See Muryama (1964).

3. Nalbandian (1971).

4. Cerami and Manning (1971).

5. For side effects resulting from cyanate administration, see Harkness and Roth (1975). Concerning extracorporeal administration, see Balcerzak et al. (1982).

6. Deliberate swelling of the red cells of hospitalized patients with sickle cell anemia by drug-induced hyponatremmia has been reported by Rosa et al. (1980). Results on the use of cetiedil are presented by Benjamin et al. (1983).

7. For a discussion of the aspirin derivatives in general see Klotz et al. (1981). The most effective, diaspirin, bis(3,5-dibromo-salicyl) fumarate, is described by Walder et al. (1980); see also Chatterjee et al. (1982).

8. The various thiol compounds studied that react with hemoglobin are described in articles by Garel et al. (1982; 1984), which include descriptions of compounds studied by earlier investigators.

9. The inhibition of sickling by nitrogen mustard was reported by Roth et al. (1972). The results with glyceraldehyde were reported by Acharya and Manning (1980). Among other aldehydes with antisickling properties are acetaldehyde (Abraham et al., 1982), 5'-deoxypyridoxal (R. E. Benesch et al., 1977), and bifunctional aldehydes (Beddell et al., 1979; Beddell, 1984). Other bifunctional agents included BME and the imidates. Results for ethacrynic acid are presented by Abraham et al. (1982); see also Schultz et al. (1962) concerning its diuretic activity.

10. A general review of antisickling compounds, with emphasis on noncovalent agents, is presented by Dean and Schechter (1978). For the results with phenylalanine and related compounds, see Noguchi and Schechter (1978) and Gorecki et al. (1980), as well as Votano et al. (1983). The studies of Poillon (1982) have emphasized the increased antisickling potency of halogenated derivatives or extended ring structures.

11. The effects of DBA (3,4-dihydro-2,2-dimethyl-2H-1-benzopyran-6-butyric acid) are reported by Ekong et al. (1978).

12. Concerning the history of quinine, see Duron-Reynals (1949).

13. Translated by the author from Pelt (1981), p. 40.

14. Aujoulat (1969); and for earlier traditions, Meyer (1984).

15. The history of the discovery of aspirin is presented by Pelt (1981).

16. Concerning the use of membrane-encapsulated drug delivery systems for sickle cell anemia, see Schwartz et al. (1983). For studies on the enhanced adhesion of SS cells to endothelial cultures, see Hebbel et al. (1980).

17. Information on the changes in the red cell membrane composition associated with sickling can be found in Lubin et al. (1981) and Franck et al. (1985).

REFERENCES

Abraham, D. J., A. S. Mehanna, and F. L. Williams. 1984. Design, synthesis, and testing of potential antisickling agents. 1. Halogenated benzyloxy and phenoxy acids. *J. Med. Chem.* 25: 1015–1017.

Abraham, E. C., M. Stallings, A. Abraham, and G. J. Garbutt. 1982. Modification of sickle hemoglobin by acetaldehyde and its effect on oxygenation, gelation, and sickling. *Biochim. Biophys. Acta* 705: 76–81.

Abrahamsson, H. 1951. *The Origin of Death: Studies in African Mythology.* Uppsala: Almquist and Wiksells.

Acharya, A. S., and J. M. Manning. 1980. Reactivity of the amino groups of carbomonoxyhemoglobin S with glyceraldehyde. *J. Biol. Chem.* 255: 1406–1412.

Achebe, C. 1969. *Things Fall Apart.* New York: Fawcett Crest.

Adachi, K., and T. Asakura. 1981. Aggregation and crystallization of hemoglobins A, S, and C. *J. Biol. Chem.* 256: 1824–1830.

Alexandre, P. 1981. *Les Africains.* Paris: Editions Lidis.

Allison, A. C. 1954. Protection afforded by sickle-cell trait against subtertian malaria infection. *Br. Med. J.* 1: 290–294.

———— 1964. Polymorphism and natural selection in human populations. *Cold Spring Harbor Symp. Quant. Biol.* 29: 137–149.

Alter, B. P. 1981. Prenatal diagnosis of hemoglobinopathies: a status report. *Lancet* ii: 1152–1155.

———— 1984. Advances in the prenatal diagnosis of hematological diseases. *Blood* 64: 329–340.

Ames, B. N. 1983. Dietary carcinogens and anticarcinogens. *Science* 221: 1256–1264.

Antonarakis, S. E., H. H. Kazazian, and S. H. Orkin. 1984. DNA polymorphism and molecular pathology of the human globin gene clusters. *Hum. Genet.* 69: 1–14.

Attah, E. G., and G. C. Ejekam. 1974. Clinicopathologic correlation in fatal malaria. *Trop. Geogr. Med.* 26: 359–362.

Aujoulat, L. P. 1969. *Santé et développement en Afrique.* Paris: A. Colin.

Balcerzak, S. P., M. R. Grever, D. E. Sing, J. N. Bishop, and M. L. Segal. 1982. Preliminary studies of continuous extracorporeal carbamylation in the treatment of sickle cell anemia. *J. Lab. Clin. Med.* 100: 345–355.

Bascom, W. 1969. *The Yoruba of Southwestern Nigeria.* New York: Holt, Rinehart and Winston.

Beddell, C. R. 1984. Designing drugs to fit a macromolecular receptor. *Chemical Soc. Reviews* 13: 279–319.

Beddell, C. R., P. J. Goodford, D. K. Stammers, and R. Wooton. 1979. Species differences in the binding of compounds designed to fit a site of known structure in adult human hemoglobin. *Br. J. Pharmacol.* 65: 535–543.

Benesch, R., R. E. Benesch, R. Edalji, and T. Suzuki. 1977. 5'-Deoxypyridoxal as a potential antisickling agent. *Proc. Natl. Acad. Sci. USA* 74: 1721–1723.

Benesch, R. E., S. Kwong, R. Benesch, and R. Edalji. 1977. Location and bond type of intermolecular contacts in the polymerization of hemoglobin S. *Nature* 269: 772–775.

Benjamin, L., C. M. Peterson, E. P. Orringer, L. R. Berkowitz, R. A. Kreisberg, V. N. Mankad, A. S. Prasad, L. M. Lewlow, and R. K. Chillar. 1983. A collaborative, double-blind, randomized study of cetiedil citrate in sickle cell crisis. *Blood* 62: 53a.

Bernard, J. 1983. *Le sang et l'histoire.* Paris: Buchet/Chastel.

Bertles, J. F., R. Rabinowitz, and J. Dobler. 1970. Hemoglobin interaction: modification of solid phase composition in the sickling phenomenon. *Science* 168: 375–377.

Bessis, M., G. Nomarski, J. P. Thiérry, and J. Breton-Gorius. 1958. Études sur la falciformation des globules rouges au microscope polarisant et au microscope électronique. *Revue d'Hematologie* 13: 249–270.

Beuzard, Y., J. Rosa, and F. Galacteros, eds. 1984. *Maladies héréditaires du globule rouge.* Paris: Doin Editeurs.

Bowen, E. S. 1964. *Return to Laughter.* Garden City, New York: Doubleday.

Browne, S. G. 1965. True ainhum: its distinctive and differentiating features. *J. Bone and Joint Surg.* 47B: 52–55.

Bunn, H. F., B. G. Forget, and H. M. Ranney. 1977. *Human Hemoglobins.* Philadelphia: W. B. Saunders.

Bunn, H. F., C. T. Noguchi, J. Hofrichter, G. P. Schechter, A. N. Schechter, and W. A. Eaton. 1982. Molecular and cellular pathogenesis of hemoglobin SC disease. *Proc. Natl. Acad. Sci. USA* 79: 7527–7531.

Bunn, H. F., and B. G. Forget. 1985. *Hemoglobin: Molecular, Genetic and Clinical Aspects.* Philadelphia: W. B. Saunders.

Bygott, J. D. 1972. Cannibalism among wild chimpanzees. *Nature* 238: 410–411.

Cardinall, A. W. 1920. *The Natives of the Northern Territories of the Gold Coast.* London: Routledge.

Caughey, W. S., ed. 1978. *Biochemical and Clinical Aspects of Hemoglobin Abnormalities.* New York: Academic.

Cavalli-Sforza, L. L., and W. F. Bodmer. 1971. *The Genetics of Human Populations.* San Francisco: W. H. Freeman.

Cerami, A., and J. M. Manning. 1971. Potassium cyanate as an inhibitor of the sickling of erythrocytes in vitro. *Proc. Natl. Acad. Sci. USA* 68: 1180–1183.

Chang, J. C., and Y. W. Kan. 1982. A sensitive new prenatal test for sickle-cell anemia. *New Eng. J. Med.* 307: 30–32.

Charache, S., G. Dover, K. Smith, C. C. Talbot, M. Moyer, and S. Boyer. 1983. Treatment of sickle cell anemia with 5-azacytidine results in increased fetal hemoglobin production and is associated with nonrandom hypomethylation of DNA around the γ-δ-β-globin gene complex. *Proc. Natl. Acad. Sci. USA* 80: 4842–4846.

Chatterjee, R., R. Y. Walder, A. Arnone, and J. A. Walder. 1982. Mechanism for the increase in solubility of deoxyhemoglobin S due to cross-linking the beta chains. *Biochemistry* 21: 5901–5909.

Chiu, D., and B. Lubin. 1979. Abnormal vitamin E and glutathione peroxidase levels in sickle cell anemia. *J. Lab. Clin. Med.* 94: 542–548.

Ciochon, R. L., and R. S. Corruccini, eds. 1983. *New Interpretations of Ape and Human Ancestry.* New York: Plenum.

Coletta, M., J. Hofrichter, F. Ferrone, and W. A. Eaton. 1982. Kinetics of sickle hemoglobin polymerization in single red cells. *Nature* 300: 194–197.

Collomb, H. 1973. The child who leaves and returns or the death of the same child. In *The Child in His Family,* ed. E. S. Anthony. New York: Wiley.

Coppens, Y. 1983. *Le singe, l'Afrique et l'homme.* Paris: Fayard.

Coursey, D. G., and C. K. Coursey. 1971. The new yam festivals of West Africa. *Anthropos* 66: 444–484.

Craik, C. S., S. R. Buchman, and S. Beychok. 1980. Characterization of globin domains: heme binding to the central exon product. *Proc. Natl. Acad. Sci. USA* 77: 1384–1388.

Crepeau, R. H., S. J. Edelstein, M. Szalay, R. E. Benesch, R. Benesch, S. Kwong, and R. Edalji. 1981. Sickle cell hemoglobin fiber structure altered by an alpha-chain mutation. *Proc. Natl. Acad. Sci. USA* 78: 1406–1410.

Das, S. K., and R. C. Nair. 1980. Superoxide dismutase, glutathione peroxidase, catalase, and lipid peroxidation of normal and sickle erythrocytes. *Br. J. Haematol.* 44: 87–92.

Dean, J., and A. N. Schechter. 1978. Sickle-cell anemia: molecular and cellular bases of therapeutic approaches. *New Eng. J. Med.* 299: 752, 804, 863.

Debrunner, H. 1959. *Witchcraft in Ghana.* Kumasi: Presbyterian Book Depot.

Delafosse, M. 1908. *Les frontières de la Côte d'Ivoire, de la Côte d'Or et du Soudan.* Paris: Masson.

Dent, D. M., S. Fataar, and A. G. Rose. 1981. Ainhum and angiodysplasia. *Lancet* ii: 396–397.

Diamond, J. 1984. DNA map of human lineage. *Nature* 310: 544.

Dickerson, R. E., and I. Geis. 1983. *Hemoglobin: Structure, Function, Evolution and Pathology.* Menlo Park, California: Benjamin/Cummings.

Diebolt, G., and J. Linhard. 1969. Hemoglobinoses et deficiencies en G6PD chez les Africans de la region de Dakar. *Bulletin de la Société Médicale d'Afrique Noir de Langue Française* 14: 65–69.

Durham, W. H. 1983. Testing the malaria hypothesis in West Africa. In *Distribution and Evolution of Hemoglobin and Globin Loci,* ed. J. E. Bowman. New York: Elsevier, pp. 45–76.

Duran-Reynals, M. L. 1949. *L'Abre de la fièvre: la prodigieuse épopée de la quinine.* Paris: Julliard.

Dykes, G., R. H. Crepeau, and S. J. Edelstein. 1978. Three-dimensional reconstruction of the fibers of sickle cell hemoglobin. *Nature* 272: 506–512.

——— 1979. Three-dimensional reconstruction of the 14-filament fibers of hemoglobin S. *J. Mol. Biol.* 130: 451–472.

Edelstein, S. J. 1971. Extensions of the allosteric model for hemoglobin. *Nature* 230: 224–227.

——— 1975. Cooperative interactions of hemoglobin. *Ann. Rev. Biochem.* 44: 209–232.

——— 1981. Molecular topology in crystals and fibers of hemoglobin S. *J. Mol. Biol.* 150: 557–575.

——— 1985. Sickle cell anemia. *Reviews of Medicinal Chemistry* 20: 247–255.

Edelstein, S. J., and R. H. Crepeau. 1979. Oblique alignment of hemoglobin S fibers in sickle cells. *J. Mol. Biol.* 134: 851–855.

Edelstein, S. J., and I. Stevenson. 1983. Sickle cell anemia and reincarnation belief in Nigeria. *Lancet* ii: 1140.

Edsall, J. T. 1972. Blood and hemoglobin: the evolution of knowledge of functional adaptation in a biochemical system. *J. Hist. Biol.* 5: 205–257.

Edwards, B. 1974. *The History, Civil and Commercial, of the British Colonies in the West Indies.* Vol. 2. London: John Stockdale.

Ekong, D. E. U., J. I. Okogun, and V. U. Enyenihl. 1978. Effects in vitro of the proposed antisickling agent DBA. *Nature* 272: 833.

Embury, S. H., A. M. Dozy, J. Miller, J. R. Davis, K. M. Kleman, H. Preisler, E. Vichinsky, W. N. Lande, B. H. Lubin, Y. W. Kan, and W. C. Mentzer. Concurrent sickle-cell anemia and alpha-thalassemia. *New Eng. J. Med.* 306: 270–274.

Evans-Pritchard, E. E. 1935. Witchcraft. *Africa* 8: 417–422.

Fabry, M. E., and R. N. Nagel. 1982. Heterogeneity of red cells in sicklers: a characteristic with practical clinical and pathophysiological implications. *Blood Cells* 8: 9–15.

Fage, J. D. 1979. *A History of Africa.* New York: Knopf.

Ferrone, F., J. Hofrichter, and W. A. Eaton. 1985. Kinetics of sickle hemoglobin polymerization. II. A double nucleation mechanism. *J. Mol. Biol.* 183: 611–631.

Finch, J. T., M. F. Perutz, J. F. Bertles, and J. Dobler. 1973. Structure of sickled erythrocytes and sickle-cell hemoglobin fibers. *Proc. Natl. Acad. Sci. USA* 70: 718–722.

Fossey, D. 1979. Development of the mountain gorilla. In *The Great Apes,* ed. D. A. Hamburg and E. R. McCown. Menlo Park, California: Benjamin/Cummings.

Franck, P. F. H., E. M. Bevers, B. H. Lubin, P. Comfurius, D. T.-Y. Chiu, J. A. F. Op den Kamp, R. F. A. Zwaal, L. L. M. van Deenen, and B. Roelofsen. 1985. Uncoupling of the membrane skeleton from the lipid bilayer: the cause of accelerated phospholipid flip-flop leading to an enhanced procoagulant activity of sickled cells. *J. Clin. Invest.* 75: 183–190.

Frazer, J. G. 1913. *The Belief in Immortality.* London: MacMillan.

Friedman, M. J., and W. Trager. 1981. The biochemistry of resistence to malaria. *Sci. Am.* 244: 154–164.

Garel, M. C., Y. Beuzard, J. Thillet, C. Domenget, J. Martin, F. Galacteros, and J. Rosa. 1982. Binding of 21 thiol reagents to human hemoglobin in solution and in intact cells. *Eur. J. Biochem.* 123: 513–519.

Garel, M. C., C. Domenget, F. Galacteros, J. Martin-Caburi, and Y. Beuzard. 1984. Inhibition of erythrocyte sickling by thiol reagents. *J. Mol. Pharm.* 26: 559–565.

Geschwind, N. 1974. *Selected Papers on Language and the Brain.* Boston: Reidel.

Gilbert, W. 1978. Why genes in pieces? *Nature* 271: 501.

———— 1981. DNA sequencing and gene structure. *Science* 214: 1305–1312.

———— 1985. Genes-in-pieces revisited. *Science* 228: 823–824.

Golenser, J., J. Miller, D. T. Spira, T. Navok, and M. Chevion. 1983. Inhibitory effect of a fava bean component on the in vitro development of *Plasmodium falciparum* in normal and glucose-6-phosphate dehydrogenase deficient erythrocytes. *Blood* 61: 507–510.

Goodall, J., A. Bandoroa, E. Bergman, C. Busse, H. Matama, E. Mpongo, A. Pierce, and D. Riss. 1979. Intercommunity interactions in the chimpanzee population of the Gombe Stream. In *The Great Apes,* ed. D. A. Hamburg and E. R. McCown. Menlo Park, California: Benjamin/Cummings.

Goodman, M., G. Braunitzer, A. Stangl, and B. Schrank. 1983. Evidence on human origins from hemoglobins of African apes. *Nature* 303: 546–548.

Goody, J. 1962. *Death, Property and the Ancestors: A Study of Mortuary Customs of the LaDagaa.* Stanford: Stanford University Press.

Goossens, M., U. Dumez, L. Kaplan, M. Lupker, C. Chabret, R. Henrion, and J. Rosa. 1983. Prenatal diagnosis of sickle-cell anemia in the first trimester. *New Eng. J. Med.* 309: 831–833.

Gorecki, M., J. R. Votano, and A. Rich. 1980. Peptide inhibitors of sickle hemoglobin: effect of hydrophobicity. *Biochemistry* 19: 1564–1568.

Gould, S. J. 1982. Darwinism and the expansion of evolutionary theory. *Science* 216: 380–387.

Greenberg, J. H. 1955. *Studies in African Linguistic Classification.* New Haven: Compass.

Gruber, H. E., K. D. Finley, R. M. Hershberg, S. S. Katzman, P. K. Laikind, J. E. Seegmiller, T. Friedmann, J. K. Yee, and D. J. Jolly. 1985. Retroviral vector-mediated gene transfer into human hematopoietic progenitor cells. *Science* 230: 1057–1061.

Hahn, E. V., and E. B. Gillespie. 1927. Sickle cell anemia. *Arc. Int. Med.* 39: 233–254.

Ham, T. H., and W. B. Castle. 1940. Relation of increased hypotonic fragility and of erythrostasis to the mechanism of hemolysis in certain anemias. *Trans. Assoc. Am. Physicians* 55: 127–132.

Harkness, D., and S. Roth. 1975. Clinical evaluation of cyanate in sickle cell anemia. *Progr. Hematol.* 9: 157–184.

Hebbel, R. P., M. A. B. Boogaerts, J. W. Eaton, and M. H. Steinberg. 1980. Erythrocyte adherence to endothelium in sickle cell anemia: possible determinant of disease severity. *New Eng. J. Med.* 302: 992–995.

Hebbel, R. P., J. W. Eaton, M. Balasingam, and M. H. Steinberg. 1982. Spontaneous oxygen radical generation by sickle erythrocytes. *J. Clin. Invest.* 70: 1253–1259.

Henderson, R. N. 1972. *The King in Every Man.* New Haven: Yale University Press.

Herrick, J. B. 1910. Peculiar elongated and sickle-shaped red blood corpuscles in a case of severe anemia. *Arch. Int. Med.* 6: 517–521.

Herskovits, M. J. 1958. *The Myth of the Negro Past.* Boston: Beacon. 1st ed., 1941.

Hibbert, C. 1982. *Africa Explored.* Harmondsworth: Penguin Books.

Higgs, D. R., B. E. Aldridge, J. Lamb, J. B. Clegg, D. J. Weatherall, R. J. Hayes, Y. Grandison, Y. Lowrie, K. P. Mason, B. E. Serjeant, and G. R. Serjeant. 1982. The interaction of alpha-thalassemia and homozygous sickle-cell disease. *New Eng. J. Med.* 306: 1441–1446.

Hobley, C. W. 1967. *Bantu Beliefs in Magic, with Particular Reference to the Kikuyu and Kamba Tribes of the Kenya Colony with some Reflections on East Africa after the War.* New York: Barnes and Noble. 1st ed., 1922.

Horton, W. A. 1979. Ectrodactyly. In *Birth Defects Compendium,* 2nd ed., ed. D. Bergsma. New York: Alan R. Liss, pp. 383–384.

Huheey, J. E., and D. L. Martin. 1975. Malaria, favism, and glucose-6-phosphate dehydrogenase deficiency. *Experientia* 31: 1145–1147.

Ingram, V. M. 1956. A specific chemical difference between the globins of normal human and sickle-cell anemia hemoglobin. *Nature* 178: 792–794.

Isichei, E. 1976. *A History of the Igbo People.* London: Macmillan.

Itani, J. 1982. La vie sociale des grandes singes. *La Recherche* 3: 744–751.

Jackson, L. C. 1981. The relationship of certain genetic traits to the incidence and intensity of malaria in Liberia, West Africa. Ph.d. diss., Cornell University.

——— 1985. Sociocultural and ethnohistorical influences on genetic diversity in Liberia. *Am. Anthro.* (in press).

Jacob, F. 1982. *The Possible and the Actual.* New York: Pantheon.

Jeffreys, A. J., and R. A. Flavell. 1977. The rabbit β-globin gene contains a large insert in the coding sequence. *Cell* 12: 1097–1108.

Johnson, F. L., A. T. Look, J. Gockerman, M. R. Ruggiero, L. Dalla-Pozza, and F. T. Billings. 1984. Bone marrow transplantation in a patient with sickle cell anemia. *New Eng. J. Med.* 311: 780–783.

Kan, Y. W., and A. M. Dozy. 1980. Evolution of the hemoglobin S and C genes in world populations. *Science* 209: 388–390.

Karp, I., and C. S. Bird, eds. 1980. *Explorations in African Systems of Thought.* Bloomington: Indiana University Press.

Kean, B. H., and H. A. Tucker. 1946. Etiologic concepts and pathologic aspects of ainhum. *Arch. Pathol.* 41: 639–644.

Klotz, I. M., D. N. Haney, and L. C. King. Rational approaches to chemotherapy: antisickling agents. *Science* 213: 724–730.

Konotey-Ahulu, F. I. D. 1973. Effect of environment on sickle cell disease in West Africa: epidemiologic and clinical considerations. In *Sickle Cell Disease,* ed. H. Abramson, J. F. Bertles, and D. L. Wethers. St. Louis: Mosby.

———— 1974. The sickle cell diseases. *Arc. Int. Med.* 133: 611–619.

———— 1982. Ethics of amniocentesis and selective abortion for sickle cell disease. *Lancet* i: 38–39.

Koshland, D. E., G. Némethy, and D. Filmer. 1966. Comparison of experimental binding data and theoretical models in proteins containing subunits. *Biochemistry* 5: 365–385.

Leaky, L. S. B., P. V. Tobais, and J. R. Napier. 1964. A new species of the genus *Homo* from Olduvai gorge. *Nature* 202: 7–9.

Lehmann, H., and C. Nwokolo. 1959. The River Niger as a barrier in the spread eastwards of hemoglobin C: a survey of the Ibo. *Nature* 183: 1587–1588.

Leis, N. B. 1982. The not-so-supernatural power of Ijaw children. In *African Religious Groups and Beliefs: Papers in Honor of William R. Bascom,* ed. S. Ottenberg. Meerut, India: Archana Publications.

Leroi-Gourhan, A. 1967. Les mains de Gargas: essai pour une étude d'ensemble. *Bull. Soc. Préhistorique Franc.* 64: 107–122.

———— 1983. *Les chasseurs de la préhistoire.* Paris: A.-M. Métailié.

Lesk, A. M., and C. Chothia. 1980. How different amino acid sequences determine similar protein structures: the structure and evolutionary dynamics of the globins. *J. Mol. Biol.* 136: 225–270.

Levi-Strauss, C. 1966. *The Savage Mind.* Chicago: University of Chicago Press.

Ley, T. J., J. DeSimone, C. Y. Noguchi, P. H. Turner, A. N. Schechter, P. Heller, and A. W. Nienhuis. 1983. 5-Azacytidine increases γ-globin synthesis and reduces the proportion of dense cells in patients with sickle cell anemia. *Blood* 62: 370–380.

Livingstone, F. B. 1973. *Data on the Abnormal Hemoglobins.* Ann Arbor: Museum of Anthropology, University of Michigan.

———— 1976. Hemoglobin history in West Africa. *Hum. Biol.* 48: 487–500.

Lubin, B. D., D. Chiu, B. Bastacky, B. Roelofson, and L. L. M. van Deenen. 1981. Abnormalities in membrane phospholipid organization in sickled erythrocytes. *J. Clin. Invest.* 67: 1643–1649.

Lwoff, A., and A. Ullmann, eds. 1979. *Origins of Molecular Biology: A Tribute to Jacques Monod.* New York: Academic Press.

Magdoff-Fairchild, B., and C. C. Chiu. 1979. X-ray diffraction of fibers and crystals of deoxygenated sickle cell hemoglobin. *Proc. Natl. Acad. Sci USA* 76: 223–226.

Mair, L. 1960. *African Marriage and Social Change.* London: Frank Cass.

Makinen, M. K., and C. W. Sigountos. 1984. Structural basis and dynamics of the fiber-to-crystal transition of sickle cell hemoglobin. *J. Mol. Biol.* 178: 439–476.

Malinowski, B. 1954. Magic, science and religion. In *Magic, Science and Religion and Other Essays*. New York: Doubleday.

Maquet, J. 1981. *Les civilisations noires*. Paris: Horizons de France.

Marx, J. L. 1985. Z-DNA: still searching for a function. *Science* 230: 794–796.

McEvedy, C. 1980. *The Penguin Atlas of African History*. Harmondsworth: Penguin.

Mears, J. G., H. M. Lachman, D. Labi, and R. L. Nagel. 1983. Alpha-thalessemia is related to prolonged survival in sickle cell anemia. *Blood* 62: 286–290.

Merlo, C. 1975. Statuettes of the Àbikú cult. *African Arts* 8: 30–35.

Meyer, P. 1984. *La révolution des médicaments*. Paris: Fayard.

Miller, D. A. 1977. Evolution of primate chromosomes. *Science* 198: 1116–1124.

Monod, J. 1968. On symmetry and functions in biological systems. In *Symmetry and Function of Biological Systems at the Macromolecular Level*, ed. A. Engstrom and B. Strandberg. Nobel Symposium no. 11. Stockholm: Almquist and Wiksell, Wiley Interscience.

———— 1971. *Chance and Necessity*. New York: Knopf.

Monod, J., J. Wyman, and J.-P. Changeux. 1965. On the nature of allosteric transitions: a plausible model. *J. Mol. Biol.* 12: 88–118.

Monteil, C. 1924. *Les Bambara du Ségou et du Kaarta*. Paris: Emile Larose.

Murayama, M. 1964. A molecular mechanism of sickled erythrocyte formation. *Nature* 202: 258–260.

Nagel, R. L., M. E. Fabry, J. Pagnier, I. Zahoun, H. Wajman, V. Baudin, and D. Labie. 1985. Two hematologically and genetically distinct forms of sickle cell anemia: the Senegal type and the Benin type. *New Eng. J. Med.* 312: 880–884.

Nagel, R., J. Johnson, R. M. Bookchin, M. C. Garel, J. Rosa, G. Schillo, H. Wajman, D. Labie, W. Moo-Penn, and O. Castro. 1980a. Beta-chain contact site in the hemoglobin S polymer. *Nature* 283: 832–834.

Nagel, R. L., C. Raventos, H. B. Tanowitz, and M. Wittner. 1980b. Effect of sodium cyanate on *Plasmodium falciparum* in vitro. *J. Parasit.* 66: 483–487.

Nalbandian, R. M. 1971. Urea treatment for sickle cell crisis. *New Eng. J. Med.* 285: 408.

Neel, J. V. 1949. The inheritance of sickle cell anemia. *Science* 110: 64–66.

Njoko, J. E. E. 1978. *A Dictionary of Igbo Names, Culture and Proverbs*. Washington, D.C.: University Press of America.

Noguchi, C. T., and A. N. Schechter. 1978. Inhibition of sickle hemoglobin gelation by amino acids and related compounds. *Biochemistry* 17: 5455–5459.

———— 1985. Sickle hemoglobin polymerization in solution and in cells. *Ann. Rev. Biophys. Chem.* 14: 239–263.

Noon, J. A. 1942. A preliminary examination of the death concepts of the Ibo. *Am. Anthro.* 44: 638–654.

Nwokolo, C. 1960. The diagnosis and management of sickle cell anemia. *W. Afr. Med. J.* 9: 194–203.

Okonji, M. O. 1970. Ogbanje, an African concept of predestination. *Afr. Scholar* 1: 1–2.

Old, J. M., R. H. Ward, K. Karagozlu, M. Petrou, B. Modell, and D. J. Weatherall. 1982. First-trimester fetal diagnosis for haemoglobinopathies. *Lancet* ii: 1414–1417.

Oliver, R., and M. Crowder, eds. 1981. *The Cambridge Encyclopedia of Africa.* Cambridge: Cambridge University Press.

Onwubalili, J. K. 1983. Sickle cell anemia: an explanation for the ancient myth of reincarnation in Nigeria. *Lancet* ii: 503–505.

Onyeama, D. 1982. *Chief Onyeama.* Enugu: Delta Publications.

Orkin, S. H., P. F. R. Little, H. H. Kazazian, and C. D. Boehm. 1982. Improved detection of the sickle mutation by DNA analysis. *New Eng. J. of Med.* 307: 32–36.

Ottenberg, S. 1959. Ibo receptivity to change. In *Continuity and Change in African Cultures,* ed. W. R. Bascom and M. J. Herskovits. Chicago: University of Chicago Press.

Overturf, G., and D. Powers. 1981. Infections in sickle cell anemia: pathogenesis and control. *Texas Reports on Medicine and Biology* 40: 283–292.

Pagnier, J., O. Dunda-Belkhodia, I. Zohoun, J. Teyssier, H. Baya, G. Jaeger, R. L. Nagel, and D. Labie. 1984. Alpha-thalassemia among sickle cell anemia patients in various African populations. *Hum. Genet.* 68: 318–319.

Pagnier, J., J. G. Mears, O. Dunda-Belkhodja, K. E. Schaefer-Rego, C. Beldjord, R. L. Nagel, and D. Labie. 1984. Evidence for the multicentric origin of the sickle cell hemoglobin gene in Africa. *Proc. Natl. Acad. Sci. USA* 81: 1771–1773.

Parrinder, G. 1951. *West African Psychology.* London: Butterworth.

Parry, N. E. 1932. *The Lakhers.* London: Macmillan.

Paterson, O. 1967. *The Sociology of Slavery.* London: McGibbon and Kee.

Pauling, L. 1934. The oxygen equilibrium of hemoglobin and its structural interpretation. *Proc. Natl. Acad. Sci. USA* 21: 186–191.

Pauling, L., and R. B. Corey. 1950. Two hydrogen bonded spiral configurations of the polypeptide chain. *J. Amer. Chem. Soc.* 72: 5349.

——— 1953. A proposed structure for the nucleic acids. *Proc. Natl. Acad. Sci. USA* 39: 84–97.

Pauling, L., H. Itano, S. J. Singer, and I. C. Wells. 1949. Sickle cell anemia: a molecular disease. *Science* 110: 543–548.

Paulme, D. 1954. *Les gens du riz.* Paris: Librarie Plon.

Pilbeam, D. 1984. The descent of hominoids and hominids. *Sci. Am.* 250: 60–69.

Pelt, J.-M. 1981. *La médecine par les plantes.* Paris: Fayard.

Perutz, M. F. 1964. The hemoglobin molecule. *Sci. Am.* 211: 64–76.

Perutz, M. F., and J. M. Mitchison. 1950. State of hemoglobin in sickle-cell anemia. *Nature* 166: 677–679.

Poillon, W. N. 1982. Noncovalent inhibitors of sickle hemoglobin gelation: effects of aryl-substituted alanines. *Biochemistry* 21: 1400–1406.

Potel, M. J., T. E. Wellems, R. J. Vassar, B. Deer, and R. Josephs. 1984. Macrofiber structure and the dynamics of sickle cell hemoglobin crystallization. *J. Mol. Biol.* 177: 819–839.

Puckett, N. N. 1975. *Black Names in America: Origin and Usage.* Boston: G. K. Hall.

Rhoda, M. D., J. Martin, Y. Blouquit, M. C. Garel, S. J. Edelstein, and J. Rosa. 1983. Sickle cell hemoglobin fiber structure strongly inhibited by the Stanleyville II mutation (alpha 78 Asn to Lys). *Biochem. Biophys. Res. Commun.* 111: 8–13.

Ringlehann, B. 1973. Immunodeficiency in sickle-cell anemia. *New Eng. J. Med.* 289: 326–327.

Rodgers, D., R. H. Crepeau, and S. J. Edelstein. 1986. Fibers of hemoglobin S: strand pairing and polarity. In *The Theory of Sickle Cell Anemia,* ed. Y. Beuzard, S. Charache, and F. Galacteros. London: INSERM-J. Libbey.

Rosa, R. M., B. E. Bierer, R. Thomas, J. S. Stoff, M. Kruskall, S. Robinson, H. F. Bunn, and F. H. Epstein. 1980. A study of induced hyponatremia in the prevention and treatment of sickle cell crises. *New Eng. J. Med.* 303: 1138–1143.

Roth, E. F., R. L. Nagel, R. M. Bookchin, and A. I. Grayzel. 1972. Nitrogen mustard: an "in vitro" inhibitor of erythrocyte sickling. *Biochem. Biophys. Res. Commun.* 48: 612–618.

Salay, A. 1966. *Les mains mutilées dans l'art préhistorique.* Toulouse: Ministère des Affairs Culturelles.

Sanger, F. 1981. Determination of nucleotide sequences in DNA. *Science* 214: 1205–1210.

Sarich, V. M., and A. C. Wilson. 1967. Immunological time scale for homonid evolution. *Science* 158: 142–148.

Schultz, R. M., E. J. Cragoe, Jr., J. B. Bicking, W. A. Bolhofer, and J. A. Sprague. 1962. Alpha beta unsaturated ketone derivatives of aryloxyacetic acids, a new class of diuretics. *J. Med. Pharm. Chem.* 5: 600–662.

Schwartz, J. H. 1984. The evolutionary relationships of man and orangutans. *Nature* 308: 501–505.

Schwartz, R. S., N. Düzgünes, D. T. Y. Chiu, and B. Lubin. 1983. Interaction of phosphatidylserine-phosphatidylcholine liposomes with sickle erythrocytes. *J. Clin. Invest.* 71: 1570–1580.

Serjeant, G. P. 1985. *Sickle Cell Disease.* Oxford: Oxford University Press.

Serjeant, G. P., and M. Y. Ashcroft. 1971. Shortening of the digits in sickle cell anemia. *Trop. Geog. Med.* 23: 341.

Shaw, T. 1978. *Nigeria: Its Archaeology and Early History.* London: Thames and Hudson.

Sibley, C. G., and J. E. Ahlquist. 1984. The phylogeny of the hominoid primates as indicated by DNA-DNA hybridization. *J. Mol. Evol.* 20: 2–15.

Siegler, P. B., ed. 1981. *The Molecular Basis of Mutant Hemoglobin Dysfunction.* New York: Elsevier/North-Holland.

Smith, F. H., and F. Spencer, eds. 1984. *The Origins of Modern Humans.* New York: Alan R. Liss.

Soyinka, W. 1981. *Aké: The Years of Childhood.* New York: Random House.

Starck, D., and B. Kummer. 1962. Zur Ontogenese des Schimpanzenschädels. *Anthrop. Anz.* 25: 204–215.

Steinberg, M. H., W. Rosenstock, M. B. Coleman, J. G. Adams, O. Platica, M. Cedeno, R. F. Rieder, J. T. Wilson, P. Milner, and S. West. 1984. Effects of thalassemia and microcytosis on the hematologic and vaso-occlusive severity of sickle cell anemia. *Blood* 63: 1353–1360.

Stent, G. S., and R. Calendar. 1978. *Molecular Genetics: An Introductory Narrative.* 2nd ed. San Francisco: W. H. Freeman.

Stetson, C. A. 1966. The state of hemoglobin in sickled erythrocytes. *J. Exp. Med.* 123: 341–346.

Stevenson, I. 1983. *Cases of the Reincarnation Type. Vol. 4, Twelve Cases in Thailand and Burma.* Charlottesville: University Press of Virginia.

Talbot, P. 1967. *Life in Southern Nigeria: The Magic, Beliefs and Customs of the Ibibio Tribe.* New York: Barnes and Noble. 1st ed., 1923.

Thomas, L.-V., and R. Luneau. 1977. *Les sages dépossédés: univers magiques d'Afrique du Nord.* Paris: Editions Robert Laffont.

Thompson, R. F. 1983. *Flash of the Spirit.* New York: Random House.

Tilghman, S. M., D. C. Tiemeier, J. G. Seidman, B. M. Peterlin, M. Sullivan, J. V. Maizel, and P. Leder. 1978. Intervening sequence of DNA identified in the structural portion of a mouse β-globin gene. *Proc. Natl. Acad. Sci. USA* 75: 725–729.

Torday, E., and T. A. Joyce. 1910. *Les Bushongo.* Brussels: Annals du Musée du Congo Belge.

Toynbee, A. 1973. *Half the World: The History and Culture of China and Japan.* New York: Holt, Rinehart and Winston.

Trager, W., and J. B. Jensen. 1976. Human malaria parasites in continuous culture. *Science* 193: 673–675.

Trowell, H. C., A. B. Raper, and H. F. Welbourn. 1957. The natural history of homozygous sickle cell disease in central Africa. *Quart. J. Med.* 26: 401–420.

Turner, V. 1965. Ritual and symbolism. In *African Systems of Thought,* ed. M. Fortes and G. Dieterlen. London: Oxford University Press.

Tylor, E. B. 1958. *Religion in Primitive Culture.* New York: Harper Torchbook. Originally published in 1871 as *Primitive Culture.*

Uchendu, V. C. 1965. *The Igbo of Southeastern Nigeria.* New York: Holt, Rinehart and Winston.

Verger, P. 1968. La société *egbé òrun* des *àbikú,* les enfants qui naissent pour mourir maintes fois. *Bull. de l'I.F.A.N.* 30, ser. B: 1448–1487.

Votano, J. R., A. Rich, J. Altman, S. Simons, and M. Wilcheck. 1983. New antisickling agents based on two aromatic moieties coupled to phenylalanine. In *Abstracts of Workshop on Development of Therapeutic Agents for Sickle Cell Disease,* ed. J. Hercules. Bethesda: NIH, p. 33.

Walder, J. A., R. Y. Walder, and A. Arnone. 1980. Development of antisickling compounds that chemically modify hemoglobin S specifically within the 2, 3-diphosphoglycerate binding site. *J. Mol. Biol.* 141: 195–216.

Wang, A. H. J., G. J. Quigley, F. J. Kolpak, J. L. Crawford, J. H. van Boom,

G. van der Marel, and A. Rich. 1979. Molecular structure of a left-handed double helical DNA fragment at atomic resolution. *Nature* 282: 680–686.

Watson, J. D., and F. H. C. Crick. 1953. Molecular structure of nucleic acids: a structure for desoxyribonucleic acid. *Nature* 171: 737–738.

Webb, G. D. 1981. Geographical mobility, status acquisition and personhood among the Awka Igbo. Ph.d. diss., University of Rochester.

Welmers, W. E. 1973. *African Language Structures.* Berkeley: University of California Press.

White, J. G. 1974. Ultrastructure features of erythrocyte and hemoglobin S sickling. *Arch. Int. Med.* 133: 545–562.

Williams, D. A., I. R. Lemischka, D. G. Nathan, and R. C. Mulligan. 1984. Introduction of new genetic material into pluripotent haematopoietic stem cells of the mouse. *Nature* 310: 476–480.

Wilson, A. C., S. S. Carlson, and T. J. White. 1977. Biochemical evolution. *Ann. Rev. Biochem.* 46: 573–639.

Wishner, B. C., K. B. Ward, E. E. Lattman, and W. E. Love. 1975. Crystal structure of sickle-cell deoxyhemoglobin at 5 Å resolution. *J. Mol. Biol.* 98: 179–194.

Yunis, J. J., and O. Prakash. 1982. The origin of man: a chromosomal pictoral legacy. *Science* 215: 1525–1529.

Zuckerkandl, E., and L. Pauling. 1962. Molecular disease, evolution, and genic diversity. In *Horizons in Biochemistry,* ed. M. Kasha and B. Pullman. New York: Academic, pp. 189–225.

INDEX

Àbikú (Yoruba), 74–77, 81

Abortion, 143–146, 152

Achebe, C., 19, 22, 66, 68

Africa: incidence of sickle cell anemia in, 1–5, 47–48, 51, 82, 152; dimensions of, 5–6; governments of, 12; and concepts of death, 17; and collision with Asia, 27, 33; health care in, 50; past populations of, 54; and prenatal diagnosis of sickle cell anemia, 144–145; and traditional medicine, 112, 160, 162. *See also* Language; Migrations

Ainhum, 83

Allison, A. C., 53–54

Allosteric mechanism, 105. *See also* Model of R and T states

Alpha helix, 110, 114

Alzheimer's disease, 114

Amino acids, 24–27, 37, 90, 96; replacement in S mutation, 93

Amniocentesis, 142–144

Ancestor worship, 13, 66–67, 83

Animism, 13, 16, 83, 90

Anopheles, 53, 60, 62

Antisickling agents: cyanate as, 60–63, 154, 155, 156; modes of action of, 110, 154–156, 168; from traditional medicine, 112, 162; identification of targets for, 115, 157–159; acting on DNA, 136–139; acting on hemoglobin, 153–160; urea as, 153–154, 156; and extracorporeal administra-

tion, 154; acting on the cell membrane, 154–155, 164; aspirin derivatives as, 158; thiol reagents as, 158, 166–168; aldehydes as, 159; nitrogen mustard as, 159; L-phenylalanine and related compounds as, 159–160; from chewing stick, 160; and targeted delivery systems, 164; acting on cell adhesion, 164; acting on DPG concentration, 165; and computer-aided design, 166–168

Aphasia, 40–41

AS individuals: probability of, 47–48; fitness of, 51; resistance to malaria of, 51–57, 60–64, 134; red blood cell sickling in, 130, 134

Aspirin, 158, 163–164

Australopithecus, 32–35, 37, 40

Awgu (Nigeria), 21, 51, 65

Bantu, 55, 82, 148

Bascom, W., 74–75

Behavior, 38. *See also* Chimpanzee; Gorilla

Biological clock, 26, 32, 36–37, 110

Birth defects, 66, 83, 86

Birthmarks, 74, 80, 83, 84, 86, 87, 175n16

Bone marrow transplant, 137, 179n1

Bowen, E. S., 8

Brain capacity, 34

Bricolage, in evolution and culture, 15, 24

Broca, P., 41